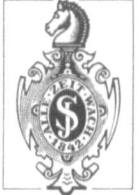

J. A. L. Bulcke A. L. Baert

Clinical and Radiological Aspects of Myopathies

CT Scanning · EMG · Radioisotopes

With 151 Figures and 30 Tables

Springer-Verlag Berlin Heidelberg GmbH

Dr. JAN A. L. BULCKE

K. U. Leuven, Department of Neurology and Neurosurgery,
Universitaire Ziekenhuizen, Kapucijnenvoer 35, B-3000 Leuven

Professor Dr. ALBERT L. BAERT

K. U. Leuven, Department of Radiology,
Universitaire Ziekenhuizen, Kapucijnenvoer 35, B-3000 Leuven

ISBN 978-3-662-02356-3   ISBN 978-3-662-02354-9 (eBook)
DOI 10.1007/978-3-662-02354-9

Library of Congress Cataloging in Publication Data. *Bulcke, J. A. L.* (Jan André Léon), 1940 –   Clinical
and radiological aspects of myopathies. Includes bibliographical references and index. 1. Neuromuscular
diseases – Diagnosis. 2. Musculoskeletal system – Radiography. I. Baert, A., 1931 – II. Title. [DNLM:
1. Muscular diseases. 2. Muscular diseases – Radiography. WE 550 B933c]   RC925.B84   1982   616.7'4075
82-10572

© by Springer-Verlag Berlin Heidelberg 1982.

Originally published by Springer-Verlag Berlin Heidelberg New York in 1982.

Softcover reprint of the hardcover 1st edition 1982

2121/3130-543210

Foreword

One of the most puzzling and striking features of many of the genetically-determined progressive neuromuscular diseases such as the spinal muscular atrophies and the muscular dystrophies is that muscular wasting and weakness in these cases is curiously selective, at least in the early stages, picking out certain skeletal muscles and sparing others. The diagnosis of these conditions has largely depended in the past upon the recognition of specific patterns of involvement of individual muscles and muscle groups, taken along with information derived from the mode of inheritance within the individual family and the results of special investigations. The investigations of most value have proved to be serum enzyme studies, electromyography and related techniques, and muscle biopsy. The advent of CT scanning has, however, introduced a new dimension; as the authors of this interesting monograph have clearly demonstrated, it is now possible, using the whole-body scanner, to define patterns of muscular atrophy in the limbs and trunk much more precisely than by any other method. Not only does this technique demonstrate which muscles are involved, but the changes in relative density provide useful information about the severity of the process and about the progress of the disease if the studies are performed serially.

This monograph is pleasantly written and most attractively illustrated. It is not, as the authors point out, a comprehensive treatise of CT scanning in neuromuscular disease; they have concentrated particularly upon their studies of a relatively limited number of conditions such as, for example, myotonic dystrophy and the Becker type of X-linked dystrophy. However, it demonstrates to the full the potential of this and other, related techniques for increasing our knowledge of the neuromuscular diseases. I am happy to recommend it to neurologists, paediatricians and radiologists alike as being a volume of very considerable interest to them in particular. But it will also be of interest to all other individuals interested in those disorders which affect voluntary muscle.

SIR JOHN WALTON

Acknowledgements

This book could obviously not have been published without the collaboration of a large number of people from many different disciplines.

All patients presented were admitted to the Department of Neurology and Neurosurgery. During their clinical investigations we were helped by fruitful discussions with our colleagues in neurology, R. VAN DEN BERGH, M.D., H. CARTON, M.D., and L. HENS, M.D. Most patients were also examined by the different members of our Study Group for Neuromuscular Diseases who helped establish and verify the diagnoses in all their phenotypical aspects. To all of them, and to the many friends and colleagues who referred patients to us, our sincerest thanks.

Many colleagues in the Department of Radiology were of substantial assistance, in particular G. WILMS, M.D., who supervised many of the scans and contributed extensively to Chapter 4 on CT scanning, while P. DE MAEYER, M.D. and L. VAN STEEN, M.D. spent many hours going over tapes and discs, selecting and recording pictures. Our thanks also to Mr. W. DESMET, Medical Photographer, who took care of most of the photography, and to the team of X-ray technicians for their skill and understanding. R. DOM, M.D., head of the Laboratory of Neuropathology, and his collaborators helped with the histopathological correlations, while J. DE MEIRSMAN, M.D. and G. CLAES, M.D. of the Department of Physical Medicine are to be thanked for their help with EMG and SFEMG and for many hours of productive talk. Also deserving of mention is A. HENDRICKX, M.D. of the Department of Internal Medicine, Nutrition Unit, School of Public Health, who carried out the fat cell and fatty acid analyses.

Special mention should be made of the willingness of R. PÁLVÖLGYI, M.D., Priv. Doz., Budapest, to contribute some of his exceptional xeroradiographs, and of the kindness of Professor Sir JOHN WALTON for writing the Foreword to the book.

Our special thanks also go to Mrs. MARIANNE BARTHOLOMEES who took unfailing care of the manuscripts. Finally, we wish to include in our acknowledgements the Springer-Verlag team for their very pleasant and efficient collaboration.

JAN A. L. BULCKE, ALBERT L. BAERT

Contents

1 Introduction

In July 1976 a 30-year-old patient presented in the Neurology Out-patient Department with a history of progressive gait disturbances since the age of 8 years. The clinical examination revealed moderate proximal muscular weakness, decreased deep tendon reflexes and above all very obvious hypertrophy of the calf muscles. His EMG was characteristic for a myopathy and serum creatine kinase was 655 U/litre (maximum normal level 55 U/litre). The tentative diagnosis was made of an X-linked pseudohypertrophic Becker-type muscular dystrophy. During the ensuing investigation we decided, out of academic curiosity one could say, to examine the patient's lower extremities by means of CT scanning. Two scans were performed, one through the thigh muscles and a second through the so-called pseudohypertrophic lower leg muscles. These scans, carried out on one of our first slow total body scanners, are shown in Fig. 1.1.

The two scans were, according to present standards, technically far from perfect, but nevertheless proved very interesting in many respects. First, we could see that the patient did not have pseudohypertrophy of the lower leg muscles, as we had expected, but real hypertrophy, homogeneous, very dense and exceeding even the size of the thigh. The thigh muscles were even more interesting. Contrary to the clinical examination, which did not reveal any muscular wasting, we found severe muscular wasting, particularly of the m. quadriceps, the mm. adductores and the hamstrings. However, at the same time more hypertrophy was found, specifically of the m. gracilis – a muscle which normally has a rather secondary function and which here, for unknown reasons, had suddenly become very prominent. The m. sartorius and the caput breve of m. biceps femoris were also selectively spared from wasting, and were probably hypertrophic as well.

These first scans, it seemed to us, immediately established CT scanning as an interesting new tool for the examination of myopathies. The discrepancies between the clinical findings in the thigh muscles and the findings on CT scanning showed that this examination could usefully be added to other clinical investigations such as EMG and muscle biopsy. The findings in both the thigh and the calf muscles stressed the potential scientific value of this examination in the study of myopathic phenomena such as pseudohypertrophy.

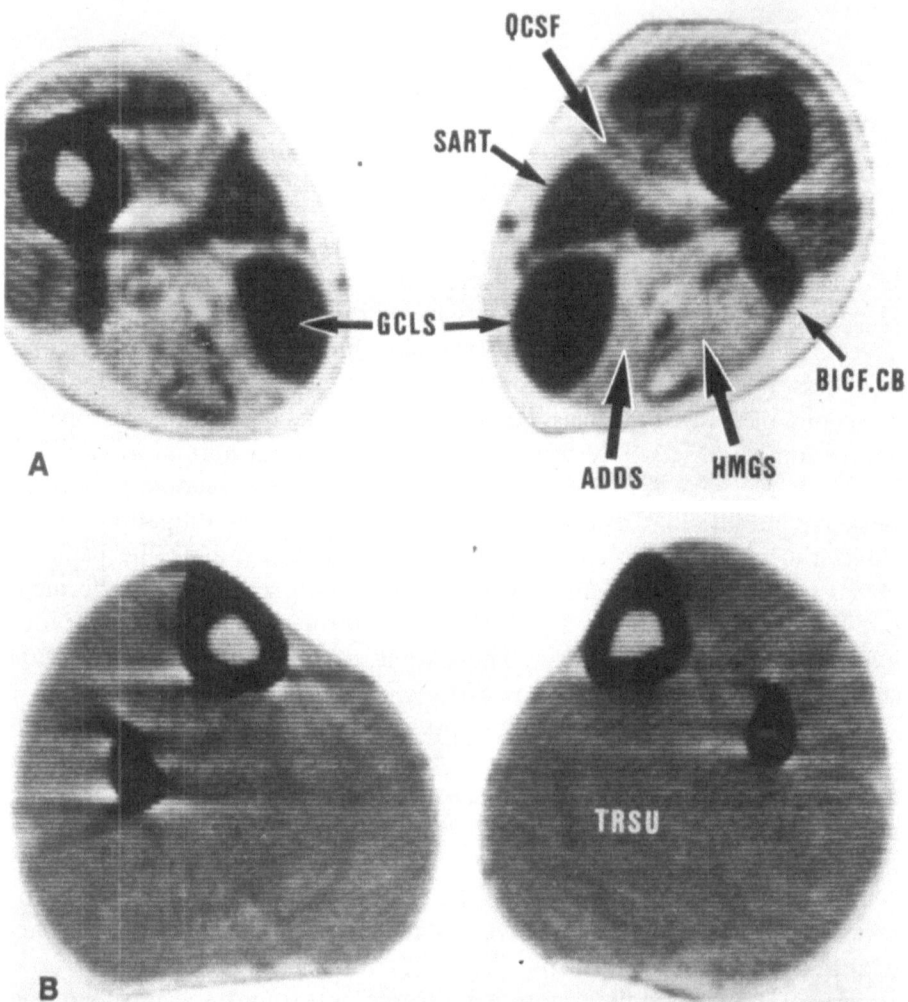

Fig. 1.1 A, B. Our first CT scan, showing the potential value of the technique.
A Atrophy of m. quadriceps femoris (*QCSF*), mm. adductores (*ADDS*) and hamstrings (*HMGS*). Hypertrophy of m. gracilis (*GCLS*) and probably also of the m. sartorius (*SART*), which is certainly well preserved. The same is true for the caput breve of m. biceps femoris (*BICF.CB*). **B** Hypertrophy of the muscles of the lower extremity and particularly of the m. triceps surae (*TRSU*)

In the following pages we provide a number of illustrations of the clinical and scientific value of CT scanning in myopathies. The main emphasis, however, will be clinical. We will try to demonstrate that CT scanning should be included in the investigation of all neuromuscular diseases because it can contribute substantially towards more precise diagnoses and more correct assessments of lesions caused by neuromuscular diseases. With this objective in mind we present (a) a description of an original standard examination procedure which can be introduced on a strictly routine basis and which produces a high yield of clinical data from a low dose of radiation and (b) a selection of CT images from some 400 scans performed during the course of investigations in patients with various myopthies.

1.1 Diagnostic Significance of CT Scanning of the Skeletal Muscular System

The most important contribution of CT to clinical medicine is undoubtedly its ability to differentiate clearly the soft tissues of the body. Conventional diagnostic radiology differentiates essentially between bone and air, as in an X-ray of the lungs (HOUNSFIELD 1980), and soft tissues such as thoracic muscles surrounding the lungs are sometimes merely seen as causes of artefacts and problems on chest radiographs (COLLINS and PAGANI 1978; GILMARTIN 1979).

The skeletal muscles constitute by far the largest soft tissue organ system of the human body, and a vast wealth of information on both their normal structure and function and on neuromuscular diseases or myopathies has been gathered, particularly during the past decade. It is therefore rather amazing that the contribution of CT scanning to the study of the skeletal muscular system and of myopathies in particular has so far remained rather limited. Several papers have been published presenting CT scanning of musculoskeletal disorders in general and especially those of neoplastic origin (BERGER and KUHN 1978; WILSON et al. 1978; GRABBE et al. 1979; HERMANN and ROSE 1979; LEVINSOHN 1980; NESBIT et al. 1981), but only a few papers have dealth specifically with the study of normal skeletal muscles (HÄGGMARK et al. 1978; WILSON 1979, BULCKE et al. 1979 a), and CT scan studies of myopathies are rare (ENZMANN et al. 1976; O'DOHERTY et al. 1977; NAIDICH et al. 1978; TROKEL and HILAL 1979; TORCH and RENO 1980).

Apart from being easy to perform, non-invasive and painless, CT scanning is invaluable as an investigation which can circumvent and solve some of the specific problems which have always hampered the clinical examination of the skeletal muscular system.

The clinical examination of the degree of muscular damage in myopathies has always been limited by several factors. Replacement by fat and connective tissue follows muscle cell destruction in many cases. This may completely compensate for the loss of muscular mass, so that even extensive muscular atrophy may escape clinical observation. The diseased muscles in

X-linked muscular dystrophies, myotonic diseases and denervated limbs may even appear hypertrophic. Moreover, the atrophied muscular mass of many patients, particularly females, is surrounded by a well-developed panniculus adiposus which either remains unaffected by their disease or increases due to immobilization. Transcutaneous appraisal of muscular damage under these conditions becomes very imprecise, and clinical instruments such as a tape measure have proven to be inappropriate. This is particularly true for muscles of the shoulder and pelvic girdles, which are usually involved early in the course of neuromuscular diseases and are therefore clinically important. Reliable correlations between the loss of muscular strength as measured by analytical muscular testing schemes and the degree of atrophy in the girdle muscles are difficult to make, because many tests of muscular strength are concerned with co-ordinated functions of several muscles rather than with the performance of individual muscles. Almost no information can be obtained about many deep-seated muscles which cannot be adequately tested for muscle strength or reached by needle EMG. By means of CT scanning, such problems can largely be eliminated. A good example is the m. psoas major, on which only very limited clinical information can be obtained unless CT scanning is performed (BREE et al. 1976; CHANG 1978; RALLS et al. 1980; KOHAUS et al. 1980; JEFFREY et al. 1980).

Besides being a powerful new problem solver, CT scanning has many practical clinical applications. By means of CT scanning muscular lesions of various aetiologies can for the first time be clearly visualized in vivo. This allows the radiologist to ascertain first of all whether lesions are indeed present, which may be useful in disputed cases of medical damage claims. However, not only can the existence of muscular lesions be verified, but their size, severity and localization, both in individual muscles or as a pattern with either proximal or distal distribution, can also be seen. Such muscular atrophy and hypertrophy patterns are known to sometimes have important diagnostic significance. A survey of all muscular lesions is also of great help in the planning of physical rehabilitation programmes, for the follow-up of the patient under treatment and for more accurate prognosis of myopathies. CT scanning has very practical applications for a better selection of suitable muscular biopsy sites, particularly for needle biopsy, and for a better interpretation of EMG results.

Careful clinical history and examination will undoubtedly remain the introduction to and the cornerstone of the examination of neuromuscular diseases, and CT scanning certainly has to be put in its proper place among other technical examinations which were introduced many years, sometimes decades ago. It is one examination among many and should be regarded as such.

1.2 Scientific Value of CT Scanning of the Skeletal Muscular System

The second objective of this book is to make clear that the radiological visualization of muscular lesions in neuromuscular diseases may also provide new insight into the nature and mechanisms of phenomena such as muscular atrophy, hypertrophy and pseudohypertrophy. It is quite clear that this examination is situated on another level of magnitude than, for example, electron microscopy; it is at almost the opposite end of the scale and makes it complete. Morphology can now be studied all the way from actual size down to the molecular level. CT scanning is an in vivo examination in which the relationships of muscular and connective tissue can be seen in their interaction with each other and in connection with nerve and blood supply. In particular the in vivo follow-up of pathological phenomena in patients may tell us more about their nature. We have tried to make a comprehensive study of basic muscular lesions and of some of the muscular dystrophies, but it seems clear to us that many findings are preliminary and that as an increasing number of cases are examined, probably with even better machines, some of these pathological phenomena will be much better understood.

Three particular points, which represent as many leads for further and probably fruitful scientific investigation, are raised by the present series of cases.

First, we will show in this study that muscular atrophy is in many cases a highly selective phenomenon; the question of how such a high degree of selectivity of muscular atrophy as this study shows can exist remains to be answered. Our first hypothesis was that this selective atrophy was based on the different fibre-type composition of various muscles. To illustrate our point we mention the work of COLLATOS et al. (1977) who examined contractile properties and fibre-type composition of flexors and extensors of the elbow joint in the cat. One could easily imagine that in a neuromuscular disease which rather selectively affects type I fibres, the muscles composed primarily of type I fibres would be affected first, while muscles primarily composed of type II fibres would be relatively spared. A situation as described in Fig. 1.2 could then be seen. The reverse could be true in diseases of the type II population. In the case of the cat the changes may possibly take place as described, but from the data now available on fibre-type composition of human muscle fibres this hypothesis does not seem to hold. Some of the data on fibre-type composition of human muscles are summarized in Table 2.1. Most muscles are mixed muscles; no fibre-type map is yet available for some, and for others, when available, the hypothesis in this simple form cannot be maintained. Other factors must be involved.

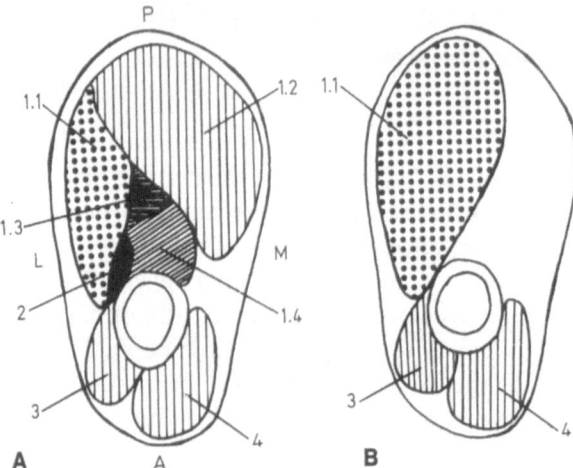

Fig. 1.2 A, B. Fibre-type distribution of type I (STO, slow-twitch-oxidative) fibres around the distal two thirds of the humerus of the cat, according to COLLATOS et al. (1977). *P*, posterior; *A*, anterior; *L*, lateral; *M*, medial. **A** *1*, m. triceps brachii; *1.1*, m. triceps, caput laterale (15%); *1.2*, m. triceps, caput longum (26%); *1.3*, m. triceps, caput mediale accessorium (79%); *1.4*, m. triceps, caput mediale intermedium (87%); *2*, m. anconeus (100%); *3*, m. brachialis (25%); *4*, m. biceps brachii (20%). **B** Hypothetical situation resulting from selective type I fibre wasting. M. anconeus, caput mediale intermedium and accessorium and caput longum have sequentially undergone atrophy. Caput laterale was spared and underwent compensatory hypertrophy. (values in parentheses: % of type I fibres)

A second phenomenon which can often be observed in the present series of cases is the rather impressive capability of the skeletal muscular system to compensate for the loss of certain muscles, parts of muscles and groups of muscles by mechanisms which are poorly understood but which can be seen as expressions of the plasticity of the system (PETTE 1980). We will present evidence to suggest that certain muscles or parts of muscles which are preserved on the CT scans are not simply remnants of the original muscles but in fact actively regenerating systems. Single-fibre EMG in some of these muscles indicates that a very active process of rebuilding is going on, characterized mainly by instability of the motor endplate potentials and an increase in the size of the motor units.

A third but least documented aspect of this study which may become increasingly important is the possibility of translating clinical impressions and clinical findings, particularly in relationship to muscular strength and atrophy, into numerical data. Obviously the present series is too small to fully exploit these numerical data in a statistically significant way, but as more and larger series of cases and longer follow-ups become available it may become possible to replace "light", "moderate" and "severe" by exact numerical values which for scientific work are much easier to manipulate.

2 Myopathies: Definitions, Clinical Presentations and Classification

Many readers of this book may not be familiar with the diagnostic vocabulary and the classification of the myopathies which we will describe. A short introduction to the rapidly expanding field of myology therefore seems indicated here. We fully realize that this is a rather hazardous undertaking. Several statements may seem over-simplified and worthy of more lengthy explanations. We therefore want to draw the attention of the more interested reader to the existence of a number of excellent recent textbooks which provide ample additional information on the subjects treated in this chapter: BOURNE 1973 a–d; ADAMS 1975; McCOMAS 1977; BETHLEM 1977; VINKEN and BRUYN 1979 a, b; JERUSALEM 1979; and WALTON 1981. In addition, descriptions of radiological changes in a number of specific diseases will be preceded by a short summary on the disease under consideration.

2.1 What Are Muscle Diseases or Myopathies?

Myopathies, in the most restricted sense, are diseases of the cross-striated muscles. Cross-striated muscles, however, are not self-supporting entities but are very dependent upon the motor neurons in the anterior horn of the spinal cord and in the brain stem nuclei for normal trophic maintenance and function. Moreover, diseases of the motor neurons can produce clinical syndromes which can be differentiated from real cross-striated muscular diseases only by means of sometimes difficult technical investigations. Some investigators have even gone so far as to claim that probably the majority of muscular diseases are induced by disturbances in the motor neurons. Because of these important nerve-muscle relationships a general consensus has developed in the literature to refer to "neuromuscular diseases" rather to "muscular diseases". Neuromuscular diseases are then defined as diseases of a functional system which is called the motor unit.

2.2 The Motor Unit

In a simplified operational concept the human motor system can be subdivided into two major subsystems. The first consists of a large but as yet un-
determined number of peripheral motor units. The second consists of an
equally unknown number of more complicated long ascending and de-
scending pathways within the central nervous system which control and co-
ordinate the functions of the motor units. Our knowledge of the anatomy
and physiology of many of these long pathways is still very fragmentary
(BRODAL 1981). The transfer of information between the two subsystems is
frequently modulated by an intricate system of interneurons.

Each of the motor units consists of four components. First, a large
neuron, usually situated within a pool or column of similar neurons either
in the anterior horn of the spinal cord or in a motor nucleus in the brain
stem. Secondly, its single axon-Schwann's cell complex which travels
through a peripheral or cranial nerve, very often together with sensory
nerves, towards one particular muscle. Thirdly, within the muscle the axon
branches out into several terminal branches which then make contacts or
junctions with a series of muscle cells. These muscle cells, connected to one
motor neuron and dispersed in the muscle between muscle cells of other
motor units, consitute the fourth component of a motor unit (Fig. 2.1).

2.3 Muscle Fibre Types

In human muscles there are essentially two types of motor units which we
can call types I and II. A type I motor unit is composed exclusively of type I
muscular cells, a type II unit of type II cells. Within the group of type II
cells a further subdivision can be made into type II A and type II B cells.
These cell types have important biochemical and physiological differences;
the biochemical differences can most easily be demonstrated by a number
of histochemical staining techniques which are now almost universally accepted (Fig. 2.2).

The ratio of type I to type II cells varies considerably between different
human muscles. Many muscles have a mixed population of the two types,
and when histochemical stains are applied to such muscles a checkerboard
pattern appears (Fig. 2.3). Some mammalian muscles, such as m. soleus and
the long muscles of the back, have predominantly type I cells and could be
called type I muscles. They contain more myoglobin, respond more slowly
to nerve signals and are very resistant to fatigue. They are adapted for long,
posture-maintaining contractions. Others contain predominantly type II

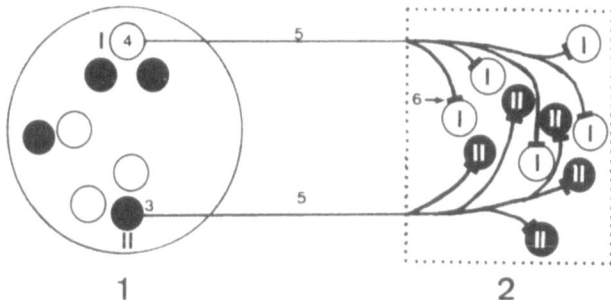

Fig. 2.1. Diagram of two motor units: (1) part of a pool of motor neurons which can be situated within either the brain stem or the spinal cord; (2) limited area within a striated muscle; (3) a type II motor neuron; (4) a type I motor neuron; (5) axons of type I and type II motor neurons connecting the neurons to a number of muscle cells dispersed in the muscle; (6) neuromuscular junction

Fig. 2.2. Biochemical and physical characteristics of muscle fibre types. *APTase,* pH 9,4, 4.6, 4.3 myosin adenosine-triphosphatase reaction after pre-incubation of biopsy in a medium of pH 9.4, pH 4.6 or pH 4.3; *NADH-TR,* NADH-tetrazolium reductase; *SDH,* succinic dehydrogenase; *α-GPDH,* α-glycerolphosphate dehydrogenase; *P'ase,* phosphatase. The fibre types described here were first described by (1) BROOKE and KAISER (1970). Other names were given by: (2) PADYKULA and GAUTHIER (1967), (3) BURKE et al. (1971), (4) PETER et al. (1972). *S (RR),* slow, very resistant to fatigue; *FR,* fast, resistant to fatigue; *FF,* fast, fatigable; *SO,* slow, oxidative; *FOG,* fast, oxidative-glycolytic; *FG,* fast, glycolytic

(1)	Type I	Type II A	Type II B
ATP'ase pH 9.4	○	●	●
pH 4.6	●	○	●
pH 4.3	●	○	○
NADH-TR	●	○	○
SDH	●	●	○
α-GPDH	○	●	●
P'ase	○	●	●
Glycogen	○	●	●
Myoglobin	●	●	○
Natural colour	dark	dark	pale
Capillary supply	high	high	low
Mitochondria	many, small	many, large	few, small
Z discs	intermediate	wider	narrower
Twitch speed	slow	fast	fast
Fatigability	resistant	resistant	sensitive
(2)	intermediate	red	white
(3)	S (RR)	FR	FF
(4)	SO	FOG	FG

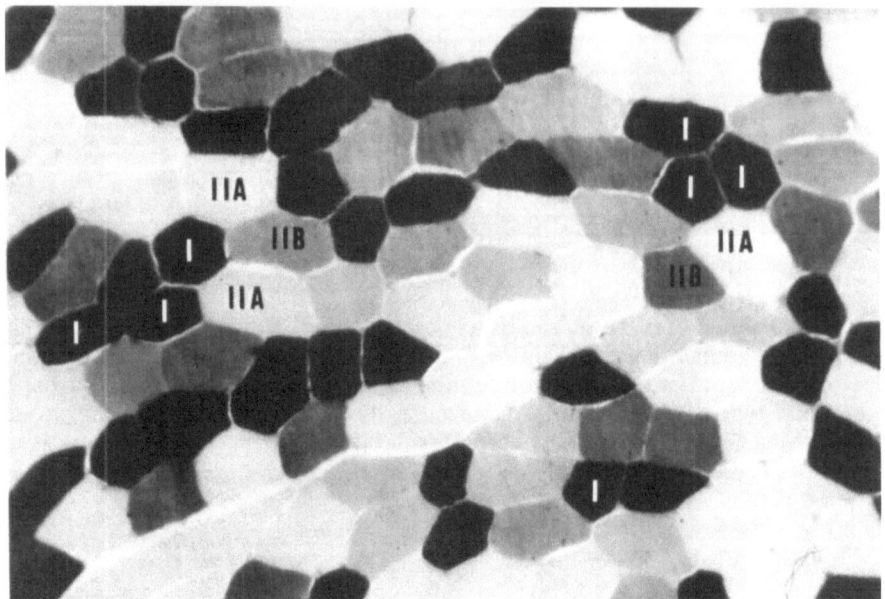

Fig. 2.3. Muscle fibre types as seen in a normal muscle biopsy. The biopsy has been histochemically stained at pH 4.6 for myosin adenosine-triphosphatase (ATPase). A checkerboard pattern appears in which the type I fibres are dark (high ATPase reaction in this pH). The type II A fibres are clear (almost no ATPase reaction at this pH) while type II B fibres have an intermediate staining

cells; these are fast-twitch muscles, specialized for fine, skilled movements such as those of the extra-ocular muscles and of the small muscles of the hand.

Motor units also have different sizes. FEINSTEIN et al. (1955) estimated that the m. rectus lateralis of the human eye contains almost 3000 motor units but only nine fibres per unit, whereas the human m. gastrocnemius, caput mediale, was found to contain only 579 motor units but 1934 fibres per unit.

As we have mentioned already, one of the important findings of CT scanning in myopathies is that muscular atrophy can be very selective, not only for certain muscles but also for parts of muscles such as deeper vs. superficial layers. As we have already discussed, the hypothesis could be put forward that this phenomenon is based on the variation in type I–II ratio in the different muscles or parts of muscles. In order to check the acceptability of this hypothesis we scanned the literature on fibre-type distribution in different muscles.

Some of the data on this subject from the literature have been summarized in Table 2.1. We have limited the description to muscles which can be seen in the standard examination procedure and have classified them in this sequence. Unfortunately, for most muscles of the body the fibre-type map is still unknown and many of the data in Table 2.1 are insufficient to allow significant statistical analysis.

At the neck muscle level only the m. sternocleidomastoideus has been sufficiently studied, and it is clear that a type II predominance exists (JOHNSON et al. 1973). The finding that in myotonic dystrophy this muscle is wasted very early in the course of the disease is therefore difficult to explain on the basis of predominant type I fibre atrophy (DUBOWITZ and BROOKE 1973), which is characteristic for this disease.

For the shoulder muscles, statistically significant differences in fibre-type distribution were found in three samples of m. deltoideus, in which there are more type II fibres in superficial layers ($P < 0.01$), and in two cases of m. pectoralis major, in which the pars clavicularis contains more type II fibres than the pars sternalis ($P < 0.05$), although the muscle as a whole has a type II predominance (JOHNSON et al. 1973). Other muscles can be considered mixed type I–II muscles with a large range of difference between the samples.

At the abdominal wall and spinal muscular level a clear predominance of type I fibres is seen in m. erector spinae as has already been explained. According to SULEMANA and SUCHENWIRTH (1972) the type I fibres are also larger than the type II fibres in m. erector spinae, their surface ratio being $1:17$.

Most of the pelvic muscles which have been examined are mixed muscles. For m. adductor magnus, however, there is a significant predominance of type I fibres in the superficial layers ($P < 0.05$) and in the deeper layers of the muscle ($P < 0.001$) (JOHNSON et al. 1973).

JOHNSON et al. (1973) also examined the relationship between type I and II fibres in superficial and deep layers of several muscles in the lower extremities. Their results are summarized in Table 2.2. The number of cases is small and certainly not enough to explain some of the selective atrophy phenomena of these muscles which we will demonstrate. However, they represent some interesting clues which should certainly be explored more extensively. In the lower extremities predominantly type I muscles would be the deeper layers of m. vastus medialis, m. biceps femoris, m. soleus, m. tibialis anterior and m. peroneus longus. In the predominantly type II group we find the superficial and lateral part of m. rectus femoris and the superficial part of m. vastus lateralis.

2.4 Atrophy and Dystrophy

Neuromuscular diseases are given different names according to the site of the defect within the motor unit (Table 2.3). Diseases of the muscles themselves are called myopathies; the defect here is situated within the muscular

Table 2.1. Fibre-type composition of normal human skeletal muscle

N	Muscle	Origin of sample[a]	Mean % Type I	Mean % Type II	Range Type I	Range Type II	No. of samples studied	Reference
1.1	m. sternocleidomastoideus	—	35.2	64.8	27.5 – 42.8	57.2 – 72.5	6	Johnson et al. (1973)
2.1	m. deltoideus	S	53.3	46.7	43.4 – 63.2	36.8 – 56.7	6	Johnson et al. (1973)
		D	61.0	39.0	46.2 – 75.7	24.2 – 53.8	6	Johnson et al. (1973)
		s	46.0	(54.0)	14.3 – 59.8	—	26	Gollnick et al. (1972)
		t	54.8	(45.2)	45.5 – 66.2	—	12	Gollnick et al. (1972)
		—	58/70[b]	5/70	—	—		Jennekens et al. (1971)
2.2	m. pectoralis major							
	Pars clavicularis	—	42.3	57.7	32.2 – 52.3	47.7 – 67.8	6	Johnson et al. (1973)
	Pars sternocostalis	—	43.1	56.9	28.5 – 57.8	42.2 – 71.5	6	Johnson et al. (1973)
2.3	m. infraspinatus	—	45.3	54.7	36.7 – 54.0	46.0 – 63.3	6	Johnson et al. (1973)
2.4	m. rhomboideus major	—	44.6	55.4	33.7 – 55.3	44.6 – 66.2	6	Johnson et al. (1973)
2.5	m. trapezius	—	53.7	46.3	32.8 – 74.6	25.4 – 67.2	6	Johnson et al. (1973)
2.6	mm. intercostales	—	65.2	34.8	—	—	31	Keens and Ianuzzo (1979)
3.1	m. erector spinae	S	58.4	41.6	33.3 – 83.5	16.5 – 66.7	6	Johnson et al. (1973)
		D	54.9	45.1	32.0 – 77.8	22.2 – 68.1	6	Johnson et al. (1973)
		—	62.5	37.5	50.0 – 75.0	25.0 – 50.0	11	Sulemana and Suchenwirth (1972)
3.2	m. rectus abdominis	—	46.1	53.9	35.4 – 56.9	43.1 – 64.6	6	Johnson et al. (1973)
3.3	Diaphragma	—	55.6	44.4	—	—	10	Khan and Khan (1978)
		—	54.9	(45.1)	—	—	31	Keens and Ianuzzo (1979)

		S/D					n	Reference
4.1	m. adductor magnus	S	53.5	46.5	41.6 – 65.4	34.6 – 58.4	6	JOHNSON et al. (1973)
		D	63.3	36.7	50.3 – 76.3	23.7 – 49.7	6	JOHNSON et al. (1973)
4.2	m. gluteus maximus	–	52.4	47.6	36.1 – 66.8	33.2 – 61.9	6	JOHNSON et al. (1973)
4.3	m. iliopsoas	–	49.2	50.8	39.5 – 58.8	41.2 – 60.5	6	JOHNSON et al. (1973)
5.1	m. quadriceps	–	50.0	50.0	33.0 – 66.0	34.0 – 66.0	24	MEYER and ELIAS (1976)
	m. rectus femoris	–	(49.5)	50.5	—	—	24	SULEMANA and SUCHENWIRTH (1972)
		S	29.5	70.5	22.0 – 37.0	63.0 – 78.0	6	JOHNSON et al. (1973)
		D	42.0	58.0	35.6 – 48.3	51.5 – 64.4	6	JOHNSON et al. (1973)
		–	13 (1)	48 (1)	—	—	8	JENNEKENS et al. (1971)
	m. vastus lateralis	S	32.7	67.3	19.6 – 45.8	54.2 – 80.4	6	JOHNSON et al. (1973)
		D	46.9	53.1	37.5 – 65.2	43.8 – 62.5	6	JOHNSON et al. (1973)
		–	56.9	(43.1)	—	—	6	EDSTROM and NYSTROM (1969)
		–	48.0	(52.0)	—	—	24	EDSTROM and EKBLOM (1972)
		–	40.0	(60.0)	—	—	26	GOLLNICK et al. (1972)
		–	57.4	(43.6)	—	—	48	GOLLNICK et al. (1972)
		–	32.0	(68.0)	—	—	6	GOLLNICK et al. (1973)
		–	50.6	(49.4)	—	—	5	GOLLNICK et al. (1974)
		–	45.7	(54.3)	—	—	55	LARSSON et al. (1978)
		–	46.4	53.6	—	—	5	PRINCE et al. (1977)
		S	30.0	70.0	—	47.0 – 89.0	15	EDGERTON et al. (1975)
		D	35.0	65.0	—	50.0 – 78.0	15	EDGERTON et al. (1975)
	m. vastus intermedius	–	42.8	57.2	34.1 – 51.5	48.5 – 65.9	6	JOHNSON et al. (1973)
		–	53.0	47.0	—	—	14	EDGERTON et al. (1975)
	m. vastus medialis	–	42.0	(58.0)	—	—	11	EDSTROM (1968)
		S	43.7	56.3	36.4 – 51.1	48.9 – 63.6	6	JOHNSON et al. (1973)
5.2	m. sartorius	–	49.6	50.4	39.6 – 59.7	40.3 – 60.4	6	JOHNSON et al. (1973)
5.3	m. gracilis	–	—	—	—	—	–	–
5.4	m. biceps femoris	–	51.0	49.0	33.0 – 69.0	31.0 – 66.0	11	SULEMANA and SUCHENWIRTH (1972)
	(caput breve)	–	66.9	33.1	56.0 – 77.8	22.2 – 44.0	6	JOHNSON et al. (1973)

Table 2.1 (continued)

N	Muscle	Origin of sample[a]	Mean % Type I	Mean % Type II	Range Type I	Type II	No. of samples studied	Reference
6.1	m. triceps surae							
	m. soleus	S	86.4	13.6	74.5 – 98.4	1.6 – 25.5	6	Johnson et al. (1973)
	m. soleus	D	89.0	11.0	80.2 – 97.9	2.1 – 19.8	6	Johnson et al. (1973)
		–	80.4	(19.6)	–	–	11	Gollnick et al. (1974)
		–	70.0	(30.0)	–	–	20	Edgerton et al. (1975)
		–	(75.0)	(25.0)	–	–	10	Khan and Khan (1978)
	m. gastrocnemius	–	60.2	39.8	–	–	6	Gollnick et al. (1974)
		–	(50.0)	(50.0)	–	–	24	Meyer and Elias (1976)
		–	56.7	32.3	–	–	10	Khan and Khan (1978)
	(caput mediale)	–	50.8	49.2	45.6 – 56.0	44.0 – 54.4	6	Johnson et al. (1973)
		–	50.0	50.0	–	–	9	Edgerton et al. (1975)
	(caput laterale)	S	43.5	56.5	37.4 – 49.6	50.4 – 62.6	6	Johnson et al. (1973)
		D	50.3	49.7	43.3 – 47.2	42.8 – 56.7	6	Johnson et al. (1973)
		–	48.0	52.0	–	–	24	Edgerton et al. (1975)
		–	52.6	(47.4)	–	–	10	Costill et al. (1976)
		–	51.0	(49.0)	–	–	11	Costill et al. (1976)
6.2	m. tibialis anterior	–	42.5	(57.5)	–	–	2	Reniers et al. (1970)
		–	56.0	(44.0)	–	–	1	Reniers et al. (1970)
		S	73.4	26.6	62.6 – 84.1	15.9 – 37.4	6	Johnson et al. (1973)
		D	72.7	27.3	67.2 – 78.1	21.9 – 32.8	6	Johnson et al. (1973)
6.3	m. peroneus longus	–	62.5	37.5	52.5 – 72.6	27.4 – 47.5	6	Johnson et al. (1973)

[a] *Abbreviations:* S, muscle sample taken superficially in the muscle; D, sample taken deep in the muscle; s, sample from sedentary person; t, sample from trained person; –, sample origin not specified

[b] Jennekens et al. (1971) studied the number of enclosed fibres of either type I or type II. Generally four or five fibres of the same kind have to be around one fibre before it can be called "enclosed". The proportion of enclosed fibres of a given type is therefore a measure of the percentage of each fibre type. In their study of 70 samples from eight mm. Deltoidei 7/70 had a rate of type I/II equal to 1

Table 2.2. Comparison of difference in type I and type II fibers in superficial (*s*) and deep (*d*) layers and lateral (*l*) and medial (*m*) parts of muscles of the lower extremities (JOHNSON et al. 1973)

N	Muscle	Difference significant: *P* at least < 0.05	Difference not significant
6	m. rectus femoris (s-d)	4	2
6	m. vastus lateralis (s-d)	3	3
6	m. vastus medialis (s-d)	4	2
6	m. gastrocnemius, caput laterale (s-d)	2	4
6	m. soleus (s-d)	1	5
6	m. tibialis anterior (s-d)	2	4
6	m. rectus femoris (1-m)	4	2
6	m. gastrocnemius (1-m)	1	5

Table 2.3. Names and definitions of neuromuscular diseases

Site of defect	Name of disease
Motor neuron	Spinal (neurogenic) muscular *atrophy*[a] (Lower) motor neuron disease [(L)MND][b]
Axon	Peripheral (axonal) neuropathy
Neuromuscular junction	Myasthenic diseases
Muscle	Myopathy (e.g. muscular *dystrophy*)[a]

[a] "Atrophy" and "dystrophy" are sometimes used erroneously as descriptive terms. Muscular atrophy can be considered a diagnosis, meaning a disease of motor neurons. In most instances, however, it is used in a more general sense as synonymous for muscular wasting. Amyotrophy is sometimes used to describe muscular atrophy of neurogenic origin. Muscular dystrophy, in contrast, is certainly never a descriptive term but suggests a diagnosis

[b] The term "lower" motor neuron indicates that it is the last or lowest motor neuron in the system

cells. The best known myopathies are the muscular dystrophies, which are genetically transmitted progressive myopathies, for which we assume one or more biochemical defects in the muscles themselves are responsible. For the large majority of the dystrophies these biochemical defects have not yet been determined. Diseases of the neuromuscular junction are called myasthenic diseases; the best known is myasthenia gravis. Diseases of the motor neurons are referred to as neurogenic or spinal muscular atrophies. Most of

Table 2.4. Outline of possible diagnoses based on predominant weakness and wasting pattern (after Walton 1981)

Muscular wasting	Muscular weakness				
	1. Generalized	2. Mainly distal	3. Mainly proximal	4. Symmetrical, highly selective[b]	5. Asymmetrical
Little or none	1.1 Polymyositis 1.2 Myasthenia gravis 1.3 Myasthenic-myopathic syndrome (Eaton-Lambert) 1.4 Periodic paralysis 1.5 Myopathy with hypothyroidism 1.6 Steroid myopathy 1.7 Myopathy with Addison's disease	2.1 UMN[a] lesions	3.1 Same as 1.1 – 1.7 3.2 Myopathy with osteomalacia 3.3 UMN lesions	4.1 Periodic paralyses	5.1 Periodic paralyses 5.2 Peripheral neuropathy 5.3 UMN lesions
Moderate to severe	1.8 M.N.D.[c] e.g. Werdnig-Hoffmann disease 1.9 Benign congenital myopathies 1.10 Polymyositis	2.2 Distal M.N.D. 2.3 Peroneal muscular atrophy 2.4 Distal myopathy	3.4 X-le and limb-girdle muscular dystrophy 3.5 Benign s.m.a. 3.6 Thyrotoxic myopathy	4.2 Ocular muscular dystrophy 4.3 Oculopharyngeal muscular dystrophy 4.4 Facioscapulo-humeral muscular dystrophy	5.4 M.N.D. 5.5 Poliomyelitis 5.6 Peripheral neuropathy

2.5 Most peripheral neuropathies

2.6 Dystrophia myotonica[d]

3.7 Glycogen-storage disease

3.8 Lipid-storage myopathy

3.9 Myasthenic-myopathic syndrome (Eaton-Lambert)

3.10 Some motor neuropathies

3.11 M.N.D.

3.12 Polymyositis

4.5 Benign s.m.a.

4.6 Thyrotoxic myopathy

4.7 M.N.D.

4.8 Motor neuropathy

4.9 Glycogen-storage disease

4.10 Poliomyelitis

5.7 Benign s.m.a.

5.8 Limb-girdle muscular dystrophy

[a] UMN: upper motor neuron
[b] Highly selective means: ocular, oculopharyngeal and facioscapulohumeral, sometimes with a highly selective component in the lower extremities (e.g. peroneal)
[c] M.N.D.: motor neuron disease, corresponds to spinal muscular atrophy at spinal level (s.m.a.)
[d] In dystrophia myotonica the weakness is semi-distal, because at the onset the forearm muscles are involved but not yet the hands
[e] x-e.: X-linked

these are also genetically determined and progressive. Here, too, the biochemical disturbances are still largely unknown.

Because it is still common usage to employ the term "myopathy" as synonymous with all diseases of the motor unit, and for instance also with such entities as myasthenia gravis, this usage has been followed in this book, although it could be argued that "myopathy" *strictu sensu* should only apply to defects in the muscle itself.

Finally, it should be remembered that neuromuscular diseases usually refer only to extrafusal muscular cells. Much less is known about diseases of intrafusal or muscular spindle cells and the same is true for smooth muscle diseases.

2.5 Making a Diagnosis

This chapter will outline how the diagnosis of a myopathy is made in a logical sequence, and in the process a number of important clinical symptoms, signs, syndromes and technical investigations will be briefly mentioned and their possible contribution to diagnosis and treatment explained.

2.5.1 Clinical Symptoms and Signs Which Raise the Suspicion of a Neuromuscular Disease

2.5.1.1 Signals from Birth, Infancy and Childhood

A significant number of myopathic patients are born as "floppy" babies (DUBOWITZ 1969). They are generally hypotonic, sometimes without real weakness but with a paucity of active movements. Some have breathing and feeding difficulties and remain in hospital far longer than other children after birth, sometimes even in an incubator.

Retardation of developmental motor milestones is the next important clue that something in the motor system is not developing normally. This is particularly significant when the parents report an important difference from other children in their family and when the gap is not closing but growing.

Finally, questions should be asked about the performance of the child in gym classes and sports. It is sometimes possible to determine quite precisely, from numerical data in the school reports, when and how fast a myopathy has manifested itself.

2.5.1.2 Something in the Family

Many neuromuscular diseases are genetically transmitted. This will often be hidden by the family or perhaps even more often ignored. Patients just do not see or are unaware of the existence of abnormalities of the motor system

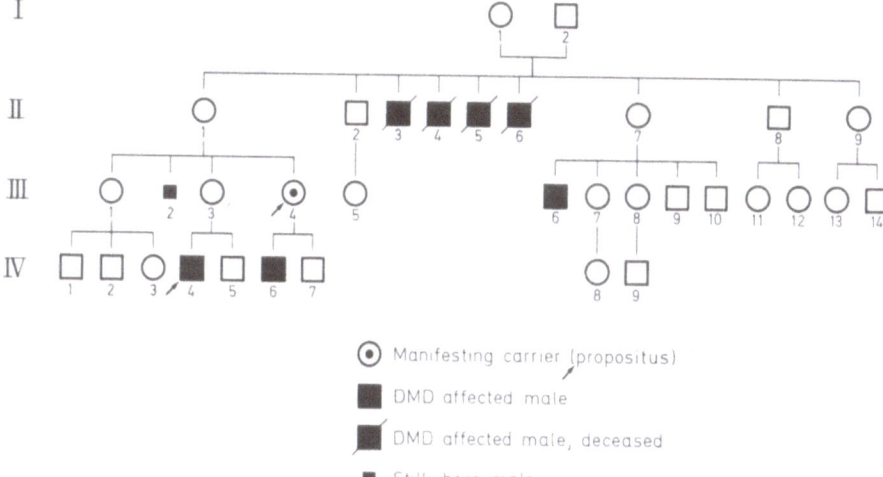

Fig. 2.4. Pedigree of a family with X-linked pseudohypertrophic muscular dystrophy of the Duchenne type (*DMD*). *Circles* represent females, *squares,* males. It is immediately apparent from this pedigree that all affected persons are males. Cases II-3, II-4, II-5 and II-6 were affected and died at early ages, probably of cardiac disease. It is also clear that the disease is further transmitted at least through females II-1, II-7, III-3 and III-4. They are called "carriers" of the disease and frequently have high CK values but no other clinical symptoms. Patient III-4, however, is a definite carrier but also has severe clinical symptoms. Such a patient is called a "manifesting carrier". Her CT scans are represented in Figs. 8.6 and 8.7. The son of her sister (case IV-4) has far-advanced Duchenne dystrophy and is shown in Fig. 8.12

in their family or even in their own life. The only solution here is to sit down with the patient and plot a pedigree of, all his known relatives, following with specific questions about each of them. In a great many cases it will soon become apparent that there is indeed "something in the family" (Fig. 2.4).

2.5.1.3 Abnormally High Serum CK Values and Strange EMG Results

Routine clinical biochemistry sometimes yields unexpected, abnormally high CK values, or strangely out-of-context EMG results suddenly appear on the chart. These should always be carefully checked before a lab error is blamed, and if confirmed they must – certainly when they occur together – raise the suspicion of neuromuscular disease.

2.5.1.4 "I Feel So Tired Lately"

Many of the initial symptoms of neuromuscular disease, in particular muscular weakness, are masked by the patient as an insidious feeling of fatigue and muscular pain which often leads to a rather sudden breakdown

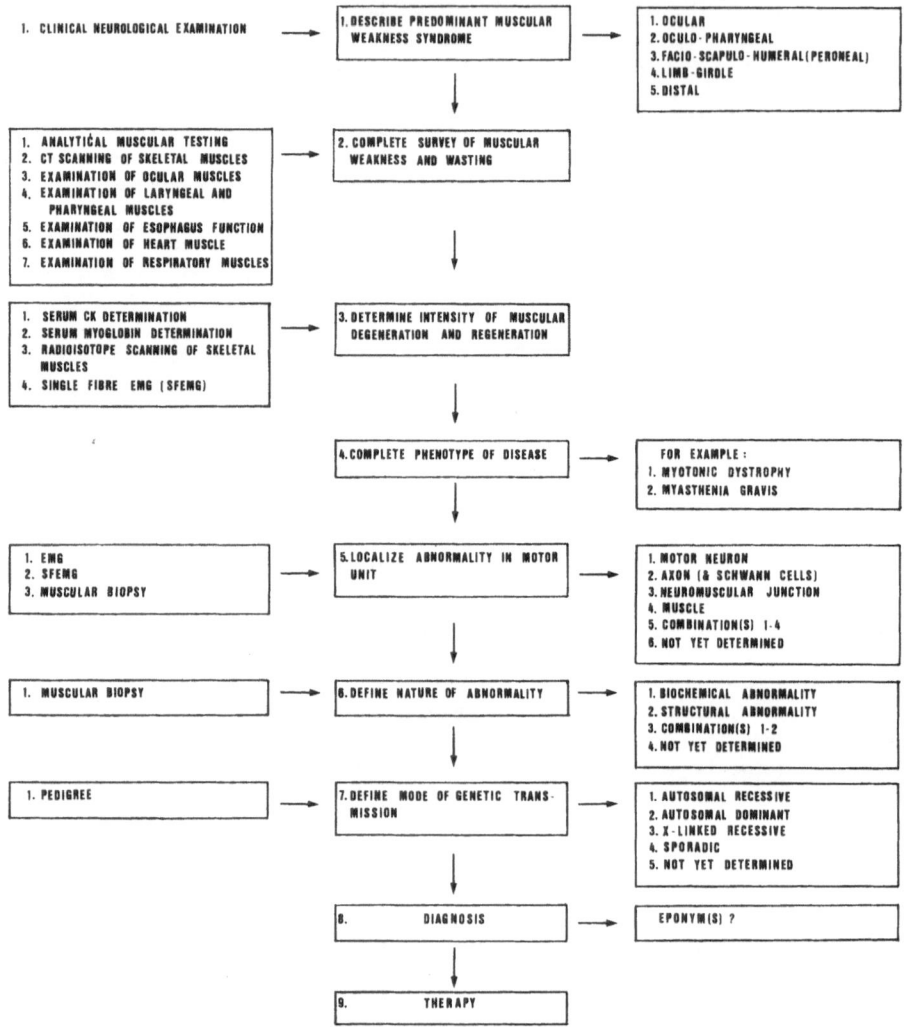

Fig. 2.5. Flow chart for the investigation of a myopathy

in work capacity. A musician will progressively feel that he is no longer able to blow the trumpet as he used to. A mechanic in a garage will suddenly have to struggle with screwdrivers and wrenches, or a hairdresser will have to reduce his appointment schedule. They may all have a facioscapulohumeral syndrome but their complaints are job-related, can easily be confused with psychological stress, and the symptoms mentioned may hide much more important weakness of muscles which they do not normally exercise.

Most other early signs such as alterations of muscular mass, spontaneous abnormal muscular movements, alterations in muscular tone and reflexes and non-muscular signs such as erythema of the face seen in polymyositis will be looked for and seen by an alert observer when such complaints are heard. If the physician persists in his efforts, a number of other signs may catch his eye, such as ptosis of the eyelids, facial diplegia, winging of the scapulae, kyphoscoliosis and hyperlordosis, calf-muscle hypertrophy and club-foot.

Finally, the physician may examine the patient further to find one of the most important data which will lead to the diagnosis of a myopathy: the description of the predominant muscular weakness syndrome. Neuromuscular diseases tend to present with weakness profiles which are different from those caused by central nervous system diseases. They are (1) eye muscle or ocular weakness, (2) oculopharyngeal weakness, (3) facioscapulohumeral weakness, (4) weakness of the proximal pelvic and shoulder girdles and (5) distal muscular weakness. Types 2 and 3 are frequently accompanied by a distal component, selective for the mm. peronei or m. tibialis anterior. Why this happens is largely unknown, but most spinal muscular atrophies, neuropathies, myasthenic diseases and muscular dystrophies follow one or more of these patterns. A limb-girdle syndrome points towards a neuromuscular disease just as a hemiparesis, a paraparesis or a Brown-Séquard syndrome points towards a central nervous system lesion. They are also nothing more than syndromes. A limb-girdle syndrome requires a differential diagnosis within the motor unit area in exactly the same way as a hemiparesis calls for a differential diagnosis within the central nervous system. One should avoid the error of moving directly from a limb-girdle syndrome to the diagnosis of a limb-girdle myopathy.

2.5.2 Admission to Hospital for Further Investigation

Once a strong suspicion of neuromuscular disease exists on the basis of information which we have described, the patient should be carefully screened to see if the diagnosis can be confirmed and further specified. This is particularly necessary to assure that no treatable diseases such as polymyositis and myasthenia gravis are overlooked, and, to carry out a survey of other muscular systems, such as the heart, the respiratory muscles and the muscles of deglutition, which may be affected together with the peripheral skeletal muscles and may be of greater danger to the patient than the peripheral weakness. In our opinion, such an investigation is best carried out after the patient has been admitted to the hospital, preferably to a multidisciplinary assessment unit. Most cases presented in this book were examined in this way.

We will now briefly discuss the various steps of the flow-chart (Fig. 2.5), outlining how such an investigation can be carried out in a logical sequence. Along the way the different investigations which are now available for establishing a diagnosis will be mentioned.

2.5.2.1 Describe the Predominant Muscular Weakness and Wasting Syndrome

The clinical examination should usually be sufficient to determine the predominant pattern of the main signs: mainly distal, mainly proximal or more highly selective; ocular, oculopharyngeal and facioscapulohumeral. The latter two sometimes have a lower-extremity selective component. When weakness and wasting are emphasized as predominant signs of a neuromuscular disease, one should certainly be aware of at least four other symptoms and signs which may either accompany them or may even at some stage of the disease become predominant, i.e. muscular pain and tenderness and muscular cramps and stiffness. It should also be stressed that clinically visible muscular hypertrophy is just as important a symptom as muscular atrophy and that all cases will eventually evolve towards more generalized muscular involvement.

Once the pattern of muscular weakness and wasting has been established, a first idea can be formed of possible diagnoses. This is summarized in Table 2.4.

2.5.2.2 Complete the Survey of Muscular Weakness and Wasting

Once the predominant syndrome is well established, two mistakes with important clinical and therapeutic consequences are often made: either one jumps directly from the syndrome to a particular diagnosis or the investigation is halted at the level of the examination of the peripheral skeletal muscles while a life-threatening defect of the heart muscle or a paralysis of the diaphragm with respiratory implications is missed. We therefore feel very strongly that a complete survey of all muscles which can be examined should be made. This is obviously a multidisciplinary effort, but if properly organized and timed it is extremely beneficial for the patient and also for the physicians who take part in these examinations; the latter gain valuable experience with myopathic patients in their particular field and can, if called upon, assist more effectively in the treatment.

Analytical muscular testing is best carried out according to the now widely accepted MRC method (M.R.C. 1943), in which the state of each muscle is recorded as follows: 0, no contraction; 1, flicker or trace of contraction; 2, active movement, gravity eliminated; 3, active movement against gravity; 4, active movement against gravity and resistance; 5, normal power.

CT scanning of the skeletal muscles finds its place right here in the investigation of a myopathy. After muscular strength has been measured, a survey of muscular lesions is carried out.

An examination of the extra-ocular muscles (EOM), especially in a purely ocular myopathy, should certainly be performed; it can then be supplemented by visual fields and evoked potentials to exclude a central nervous system disorder. A slit-lamp examination to detect cataract in myotonic dystrophy, pupillometry in the follow-up of medication in patients with myasthenia gravis and electroretinography to look for degeneration of the retina as in the Kearns and Sayre syndrome (see Sect. 2.5.2.4) can also be requested. Although in myasthenia gravis an edrophonium (Tensilon, Roche) test is frequently carried out to demonstrate that ptosis improves, changes in the bulbar muscles should be looked for instead. Ocular muscles may still be normal or underdosed while bulbar and respiratory muscles may already be overdosed. A positive Tensilon test in a cholinergic-weakness syndrome could therefore lead to erroneous therapeutic reactions.

Examination of laryngeal and pharyngeal muscles should be performed by the ENT specialist. In addition to the clinical examination, EMG of the velum palatinum and of m. cricothyroideus can be performed, together with stapedometry, m. stapedius being perhaps the smallest striated muscle of the body which can be examined.

Examination of the oesophageal function must be performed, particularly when complaints of dysphagia with inherent danger of aspiration pneumonia are present. The upper part of the oesophagus, which consists of striated muscle, can be examined, although sometimes with great difficulty, by EMG, while examination of the lower part can more easily be performed by oesophagus manometry or contrast radiography.

Examination of the heart musculature should be considered obligatory in all neuromuscular diseases. After the clinical examination, an ECG, an echocardiogram and a phonocardiogram must be made. All too often life-threatening and easily recognizable disorders are missed, with catastrophic consequences. The same is true for the respiratory muscles. Measurements of pulmonary volume and pressure changes, gas exchange parameters and radioscopy of the diaphragm should always be recorded.

2.5.2.3 Determine the Intensity of Muscular Degeneration and Regeneration

The determination of serum CK is undoubtedly the most important single parameter of the intensity of muscular destruction. To be totally sure that one is dealing with muscular CK, an electrophoretic or immunological analysis of the serum should be included so that the relative amount of muscle (MM) and heart (MB) isoenzyme can be ascertained. Next to creatine kinase, serum myoglobin determination by radio-immunoassay is probably the best single parameter of muscular degeneration. Radio-isotope scanning of skeletal muscles is an excellent method of localizing the main areas of generalized or regional muscular destruction. This is explained in Chap. 3.

The regenerative activity of skeletal muscles is characterized by an increase in the size or fibre density of the motor units and by an important instability of motor end-plates. These are the parameters for which single-fibre EMG is perfectly suitable. Follow-up of SFEMG results, particularly in areas which are under visual control by CT scanning, can provide very valuable information on the regenerative capacities of diseased muscle.

2.5.2.4 Complete the Phenotype of the Disease

In several diseases the disorder of the skeletal muscles is only one of the phenotypical features. Two examples, myotonic dystrophy and the Kearns and Sayre syndrome, will be mentioned here.

One could say that dystrophia myotonica is not a neuromuscular but a rather generalized disease in which the skeletal muscles are also involved. The disease is, however, characterized by important endocrine disturbances, cataract, immunological abnormalities such as high IgG catabolism and many other features, some of which will be described in more detail in Chap. 7. Some members of families with myotonic dystrophy have the full phenotype, others have only minor features, such as cataract.

The Kearns and Sayre syndrome is an ocular myopathy plus (therefore sometimes called "ophthalmoplegia plus") a number of other features including pigmentary degeneration of the retina, cardiomyopathy, growth failure, nerve deafness, ataxia, dementia and a raised cerebrospinal fluid protein level. A non-systematic approach in which the investigation is halted once the ptosis and ophthalmoplegia have been described will never be able to reach this diagnosis.

2.5.2.5 Localize the Abnormality in the Motor Unit

Once the clinical picture has been fully described, more precise diagnostic data are required. The first is the localization of the abnormality within the motor unit. Besides the clinical examination, which has probably already given some clues, EMG and muscular biopsy are important. In the EMG examination certain patterns at rest and during contraction are quite specific for each localization in the motor unit. SFEMG has become one of the most interesting examinations of the function of the neuromuscular junction.

All patients with a myopathy should have a muscle biopsy. Certain patterns, particularly of histochemical staining, such as grouping of type I and II fibres as a consequence of axonal sprouting, are characteristic for a neurogenic disorder. Others, such as large variation in fibre diameter, are more characteristic for a myopathy.

2.5.2.6 Define the Nature of the Abnormality

A muscle biopsy is mandatory, particularly to define the nature of the abnormality in a true myopathy. In many cases, particularly of muscular dystrophies, the defect will remain obscure despite extensive investigations. In some cases one will be able to come closer to a diagnosis, however, either by the description of structural abnormalities (for instance in the mitochondria), or in a few cases by proving an enzyme defect in the biochemical investigation of the biopsy material.

2.5.2.7 Define the Mode of Genetic Transmission

As we have already stated, the only way to obtain this information is to draw up a pedigree and to examine as many members of the family as possible.

2.5.2.8 The Diagnosis

Once all the steps described have been taken, one should be able to formulate a diagnosis. The degree of accuracy will depend fully on the amount of information one has been able to gather in the previous steps. A limb-girdle syndrome of mild muscular weakness, without serious muscular wasting, with rather low intensity of degeneration, with the defect localized in muscle and absence of muscle phosphorylase, and which is genetically transmitted as an autosomal recessive trait, permits a very precise diagnosis of McArdle's disease. A limb-girdle syndrome with severe weakness and important wasting, with a high degree of muscular degenerative activity, with the defect localized in muscle and characterized by important inflammatory infiltrate and sporadic incidence is undoubtedly polymyositis.

Eponyms can be confusing. Although it is impossible to read the current literature on myopathies without knowing the meaning of, for example, Becker's disease, they should be avoided wherever a scientific term can be used instead.

2.5.2.9 Therapy

Myopathies have the reputation of being untreatable. This is not true for a growing number of them, in particular for myasthenia gravis and polymyositis, which can even be called curable. But it is certainly true that better methods of treatment are needed for most neuromuscular diseases.

3 Conventional Radiological Techniques and Radioisotope Methods in the Investigation of Myopathies

Prior to and independent of the introduction of CT into clinical medicine, diagnostic radiology and nuclear medicine made significant contributions to the study of diseases involving the neuromuscular system. Many of these procedures will continue to be employed and further developed, either separately or integrated with others such as CT and ultrasound (KOROBKIN 1978). Therefore a description of them seems indicated here.

Many diseases have been described in which the muscular and the skeletal system are both affected. They include a number of hereditary syndromes or birth defects in which the musculoskeletal symptomatology constitutes a more or less important part of the total clinical syndrome, and in which the demonstration by the radiologist of the skeletal abnormalities adds valuable information to the diagnostic process. On the other hand, several methods have been elaborated to demonstrate changes within the muscles themselves. They include soft tissue radiography, xeroradiography and radioisotope techniques.

3.1 Birth Defects with Musculoskeletal Involvement

MCKUSICK (1978) and BERGSMA (1979) describe approximately 50 birth defects which may involve both the skeletal and the muscular system; several more are described in the literature (GAY and KUHN 1976; SPRANGER et al. 1980). Many of these syndromes are very rare. They are mostly multi-system disorders and the relative importance of the myopathic and skeletal features is very variable and often rather limited. In most cases the diagnosis is made at birth or in early infancy. The predominant muscular symptom is hypotonia, producing a floppy baby syndrome (DUBOWITZ 1969), sometimes followed by muscular hypertonia when the CNS is involved. The radiological features of the skeletal system are limited at that age because its development is not yet completed. The radiological signs most frequently encountered include: micro-, macro-, brachy- and scaphocephaly, abnormally tall or short stature, kyphosis, scoliosis and kyphoscoliosis, lordosis, and poly-, brachy- and syndactylia. The radiological abnormalities should be looked for, but in only a minority of cases do they belong to the minimal diagnostic criteria.

The diversity of the relationships between skeletal and muscular signs in the group of birth defects is clearly illustrated in the autosomal dominant and recessive syndromes of arthrogryposis (multiplex congenita, AMC), the main features of which are summarized in Table 3.1. As can be seen AMC can represent at least five different aetiologies and although the skeletal abnormalities are essentially the same, the myopathic symptoms and signs are very different. In type 1 the muscular atrophy around the affected joints is presumed to be either of neurogenic origin or due to disuse. It may eventually progress, together with the underlying pathology. In type 2 essentially disuse atrophy is to be found. In the third and most common type all signs are essentially neurogenic. As the cerebral atrophy progresses spasticity also appears. In the fourth type the muscles may initially be hypotrophic, but without either neurogenic or myogenic features. The fifth, and most controversial type shows signs of an arrested, burned out myopathy. Some of these myopathic forms of AMC have been described as separate entities such als Ullrich's disease. NIHEI et al. (1979) described 15 cases of this syndrome, which consists of proximal joint contractures, muscular hypotonia, prominent calcaneus, high arched palate and normal intelligence. Some muscular dystrophies can also be considered part of this group of hereditary diseases and in some of them the skeletal abnormalities are an important part of the diagnosis. This is particularly the case in myotonic diseases. Chondrodystrophic myotonia, described by SCHWARTZ and JAMPEL (1962) and well documented since then (CAO et al. 1978), is characterized by myotonia, unusual ocular and facial abnormalities together with radiological abnormalities such as high arched palate, thoracolumbar lordosis or kyphoscoliosis, hip dysplasia, retardation of bone age and short stature. In myotonic dystrophy the skeletal abnormalities are more subtle but not less important. They include a small sella turcica, possibly in relation to the widespread endocrinological abnormalities, and hyperostosis of the skull vault (CAUGHEY 1952).

In other muscular dystrophies, too, skeletal abnormalities are well known. WALTON and WARRICK (1954) described osseous changes in Duchenne muscular dystrophy. They start with narrowing of the shafts and rarefaction of the epiphyses of the long bones. The development of the flat bones is impaired and coxa valga is frequently seen. At later stages severe kyphoscoliosis usually occurs, or more seldom a long thoracolumbar lordosis (WILKINS and GIBSON 1976). Widespread decalcification and disorganization of the skeletal system are responsible for easy fracturing. WALTON and WARRICK (1954) tried to demonstrate that the bone changes are secondary to the myopathy, and not due to a common cause as in many of

Table 3.1. Arthrogryposis (multiplex congenita, AMC)

Minimal diagnostic criteria (MDC), pathogenesis	Muscular signs	Skeletal signs
Non-progressive limitation of joint movement in at least two sites, present at birth (FISHER et al. 1970)		
AMC can be:		
1. The first syndrome of a number of a etiologically well-defined disease entities: trisomy 18, Potter's syndrome, meningomyelocele, dwarfism, etc.	Muscular atrophy around affected joints	Scoliosis, abnormal carpal and tarsal bones, (cleft palate)
2. Produced by any environmental factor causing decreased movement in utero, e.g. space limation, drugs, infection (WYNNE-DAVIES and LLOYD-ROBERTS 1976)	Muscular atrophy around affected joints	Scoliosis, abnormal carpal and tarsal bones
3. Due to loss of anterior horn cells (neurogenic origin). Neurogenic basis is most common cause of AMC (BARUCHA et al. 1972). This form may be associated with cerebral and optic atrophy and microcephaly (FRISCHKNECHT et al. 1960) AD or AR.[a]	Muscular atrophy around affected joints, "neurogenic" EMG pattern	Scoliosis, abnormal carpal and tarsal bones, (microcephaly)
4. Due to primary failure of muscle embryogenesis; AD or AR	Muscular hypotonia, hypotrophy and fibrosis	Scoliosis, abnormal carpal and tarsal bones
5. Due to congenital non-progressive myopathy (PEARSON and FOWLER 1963) [is controversial (DASTUR et al. 1972)]; AD or AR	Muscular atrophy around affected joints, "myogenic" EMG pattern, CK[b] elevated	Scoliosis, abnormal carpal and tarsal bones

[a] AD or AR, autosomal dominant or autosomal recessive
[b] CK, creatine kinase

the birth defects described previously. Skeletal changes, however, can also be responsible for myopathic symptoms. This is demonstrated by the hypotonia which accompanies osteogenesis imperfecta (DUBOWITZ 1969), and in which the muscular symptoms are secondary to the bone changes.

A peculiar myopathy is known to occur in association with skeletal osteomalacia due to hyperparathyroidism or vitamin D deficiency. Parathyroid hormone has several functions. It mobilizes calcium from bone, increases reabsorption of calcium and excretion of phosphate in the kidney and stimulates the renal conversion of 25-hydroxycholecalciferol to 1.25 dihydroxycholecalciferol, a potent vitamin D which in turn facilitates intestinal absorption of calcium and its incorporation in bone (HAUSSLER and McCAIN 1977; HABENER and POTTS 1978). This vitamin D also acts on muscle. It augments sarcoplasmic reticulum and mitochondrial calcium uptake, and protein and ATP synthesis (PLEASURE et al. 1979). Primary and secondary hyperparathyroidism and vitamin D deficiency will lead to generalized skeletal osteomalacia, but will also affect muscle. The calcium disturbances will result in a proximal myopathy with muscle weakness, atrophy and myalgia (SCHOTT and WILLS 1975).

3.2 Soft Tissue Radiography

The high permeability of soft tissues to conventional X-rays prevents detailed examination of muscular tissue. The projected shadows of the muscles are usually poorly outlined, homogeneous and give no information about internal structure. In a number of pathological conditions, however, calcium accumulates within muscular lesions so that they do become visible on standard radiographs. On the other hand, by using softer X-rays and fine-grain film, improvements can be obtained so that skin, subcutaneous tissue, muscular fascia, blood vessels and intramuscular density changes which are due to disease can be recognized.

3.2.1 Calcified Muscular Lesions

Calcified muscular lesions can be subdivided into two main groups: one in which amorphous calcium is deposited within the muscles in the absence of osteoblastic activity and a second in which calcium apatite crystals are incorporated in newly formed bone tissue within the muscles. The latter condition has been described in the literature under several names, such as neurogenic ossifying fibromyopathy (SOULE 1945), neurogenic osteoma (BENASSY 1966) and myositis ossificans (MILLER and O'NEILL 1949). Such names are misleading because they suggest a non-proven neurogenic aetiology or an inflammatory origin which does not seem to be present (ADAMS 1975). More "neutral" names such as soft tissue ossification (ABRAMSON 1948), heterotopic ossification (DAMANSKY 1961) and particularly ectopic ossification (KEWALRAMANI 1977) seem better suited to describe this disease, which may be either hereditary or acquired.

Hereditary ectopic ossification [or hereditary myositis ossificans progressiva (AKIN et al. 1975)] seems to be transmitted as an autosomal dominant trait (EATON et al. 1957; TÜNTE et al. 1967; LETTS 1968). Almost all cases described in the literature occur in children and young adults. The syndrome usually starts as a painless swelling of the neck and the back muscles, sometimes with a torticollis syndrome. The swollen muscles indurate progressively as ectopic calcification continues. After a number of years most of the skeletal muscular system in affected, particularly the neck, the back and the limb girdles, together with their tendons and fascia. Although frequently painless, the ossifications can become tender and the patient may have accompanying fever, mimicking acute rheumatism. The bones can eventually become deformed by the ossified muscles. Involvement of respiratory muscles can lead to pulmonary complications which are the main cause of death. Steroids and a pyrophosphate analogue called diphosphonate have been recommended as treatment (WEISS et al. 1971; RUSSELL et al. 1969). Diphosphonate has been known for many years to play a role in calcium homoeostasis (RUSSELL et al. 1970).

Not all hereditary cases have the same malignant course. Some may develop, without antecedent trauma, towards circumscribed deposits of ectopic bone within a limited number of muscles. If they proliferate rapidly, however, they may be mistaken for sarcomas (OGILVIE-HARRIS et al. 1980).

Sporadic ectopic ossifications are seen either in relation to trauma or to CNS and neuromuscular disorders. An injury to muscle will almost always heal spontaneously without sequelae. In a very limited number of cases, however, the trauma is followed a few weeks later by muscle stiffness and a painful calcification at the site of the injury (ACKERMAN 1958; ELLIS and FRANK 1966). In certain professions and sports, some individuals may develop similar ossifications in over-exercised muscles: "rider's bone" in the m. adductor longus of horse-riders, "drill bone" in m. pectoralis and m. deltoideus and ossifications in m. biceps, m. brachialis, m. brachioradialis and m. biceps femoris in athletes (JONES and WARD 1980). Ectopic ossifications are also seen in chronic nervous diseases, perhaps most often in the pelvic, thigh and knee muscles of traumatic paraplegics. A disturbance of the paravertebral venous plexus has been postulated as the cause (MAJOR et al. 1980; SEIGEL 1980). How far such sporadic cases of ectopic ossification are either truly acquired or hereditary is not clear. A predisposing hereditary factor can be suspected, because several attempts to reproduce the process in animals have been unsuccessful (TWEEDAALE et al. 1957).

Calcification of muscle due to the deposition of amorphous calcium in the absence of osteoblastic activity can be metastatic, in conjunction with abnormalities of calcium and phosphate metabolism due to vitamin D deficiency and/or parathyroid dysfunction, tumoral calcinosis, milk-alkali syndrome and chronic renal failure. Such calcium deposits are also present in many conditions which cause muscular necrosis, such as muscular dystrophies. In Duchenne muscular dystrophy, tiny focal areas of necrosis containing high calcium concentrations are one of the earliest findings. These lesions, however, cannot be visualized by X-ray. Radioisotope techniques are much more suitable for this purpose. Only after intramuscular injections (KEATS 1978), in systemic lupus erythematosus (BUDIN and FELDMAN 1975), in diabetes (CAMPBELL and FELDMAN 1975) and in calcific tendinitis of the neck (NEWARK et al. 1978), in which the necrotic lesions are larger, can they be seen.

3.2.2 Soft X-rays

Several radiologists have tried in the past to adopt classic high-kV clinical radiology to detailed examination of skeletal muscles by adding filtering screens, altering focusing distances and exposure times, changing films, and modifying development and reproduction procedures (ALLEN and CALDER 1940; MELOT 1941; PONS 1958; NEMOURS-AUGUSTE 1959). The results of these experiments have not been very successful.

A more useful line of investigation, this time with low-kV techniques, started with the systematic work of FRANTZELL (1951), FRANTZELL and INGELMARK (1951) and FRANTZELL et al. (1952).

FRANTZELL and INGELMARK (1951) examined 222 healthy persons of different ages and stressed the fact that fat is the constituent on which soft tissue radiography should concentrate. They described the four essential locations of fat tissue as subcutaneous, interfascicular or perimysial, subfascicular and endomysial or interstitial. They demonstrated that in neuromuscular disease, linear striations are seen in the muscles which are localized in the perimysial fat; they considered this to be the only compartment of interest in neuromuscular disease. The increase in fat content of the muscles, from almost 0% in 20-year-old males to up to 85% in 65-year-old females was found to be localized mainly in the other compartments.

A few years later, DI CHIRO and NELSON (1965) used essentially the same approach to study the histological correlations of the radiological findings on soft tissues of the extremities in a number of neuromuscular diseases. They emphasized that good photographic reproduction of soft X-rays was very important, and often more satisfactory that the original film. They also described disappointing results in the use of water-soluble contrast media to enhance, muscular contrast. They found that in healthy young persons the normal musculature is compact and homogeneous. Age and obesity, castration and immobilization (INGELMARK and HELANDER 1951) were found to increase the subcutaneous, intermuscular and subfascial fat which increased the delineation of the individual muscles, while the interstitial fat remained normal under these conditions. They found that in patients over 40 years of age a less orderly, blotchy fat infiltration was found which was roentgenologically distinct from and more fequent than the linear streaks seen in patients with progressive muscular dystrophy. The linear fat streaks were found to be always abnormal in patients, below the age of 30. They could not find any significant difference between the fat striations observed in various forms of spinal muscular atrophy and myopathy. Only in progressive pseudohypertrophic muscular dystrophy did they find that the particularly neat pattern of fine parallel and straight striations, best seen in the calves but also in the thigh, and making the muscles resemble fish flesh, might be of diagnostic significance.

By comparing biopsy and radiological muscular findings they concluded that 56% of the biopsies of these muscles the correlation between the degree of fat estimated by radiology and that found histologically was very precise, varying to only a small degree in 92% of the cases. They also confirmed that the fat content increased with increasing severity of the disease. They found, however, that biopsy corresponded more closely to the clinical involvement than did radiology. Clinical severity was also often found to be greater than was indicated by either soft tissue radiography or biopsy estimates of fat content. They found soft tissue radiography with fat infiltration estimates totally unreliable below the age of 5 or 6 years, and particularly in the group of floppy babies.

More recently PÁLVÖLGYI (1978) made a new study of the basic radiological findings by soft tissue radiography of the limb muscles in healthy persons and in different neuromuscular diseases (Figs. 3.1, 3.2). He, too, found that in healthy young persons individual muscles can never be delineated, except for those of the forearm, and that other structural elements such as fascia, nerves and blood vessels cannot be seen. Normal muscles are smooth, rounded and homogeneous, and very symmetrical in appearance and size. Even a few millimetres of difference in size is considered abnormal. Muscular atrophy was found to be characterized by linear streaks of fat within the muscles. This is always abnormal below the age of 30 but very frequent above 65 years. The author confirmed this inability to distinguish between neurogenic atrophy and myopathy, and that the pattern already described by DI CHIRO and NELSON (1965) for pseudohypertrophic muscular dystrophy is specific and diagnostic for this disease. A similar comprehensive study was carried out 2 years later by PÁLVÖLGYI and GALLAI (1980) in which they drew attention to the selectivity of muscular atrophy in various diseases. They observed selective areas of atrophy within in-

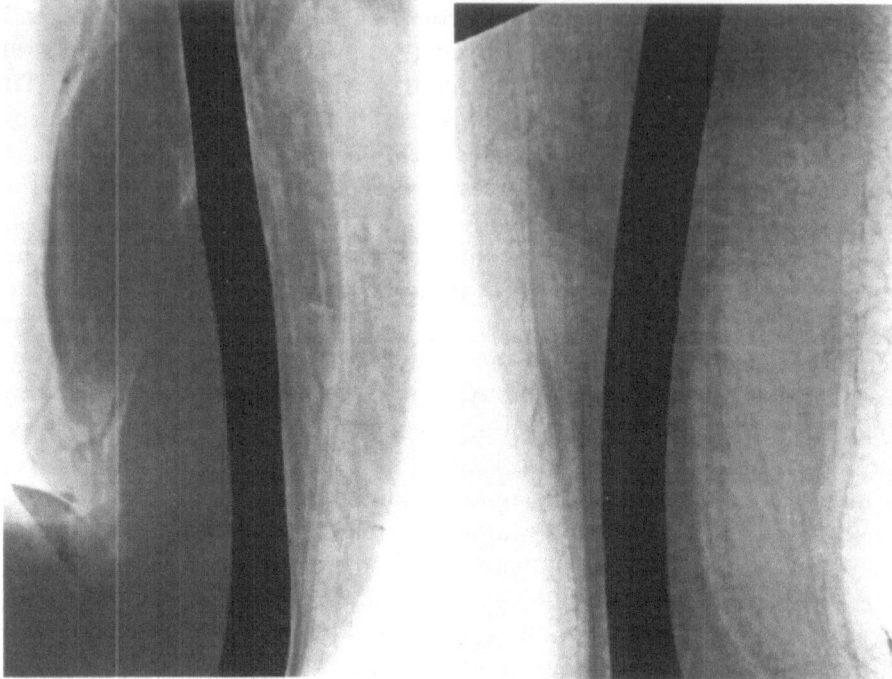

Fig. 3.1   **Fig. 3.2**

Fig. 3.1. Lateral soft tissue radiography of skeletal muscles of the upper arm with post-poliomyelitic lesions. The flexors of the upper arm, m. biceps brachii and m. brachialis are well preserved and hypertrophic. The m. triceps brachii shows moderate striation and atrophy. The subcutis of the m. triceps brachii is markedly thicker than that of the m. biceps brachii. (Courtesy of R. PÁLVÖLGYI, M. D., Priv. Doz.)

Fig. 3.2. Lateral view of thigh muscles of patient with progressive muscular dystrophy. The musculature is almost completely destroyed and replaced by fat tissue. Only the outline of m. quadriceps femoris is still visible. (Courtesy of R. PÁLVÖLGYI, M. D., Priv. Doz.)

dividual muscles, selective atrophy of specific muscles and muscle groups and asymmetry between two identical but contralateral muscles. No explanation for this phenomenon could be given. Other studies by the same author have described soft tissue X-ray findings in muscular pseudo-hypertrophy (PÁLVÖLGYI and GALLAI 1979), anterior horn cell lesions (PÁLVÖLGYI 1979), closed muscle and tendon injuries of the upper arm (PÁLVÖLGYI and BÁLINT 1979) and lacerations in tendons and muscles in the Ehlers-Danlos syndrome (PÁLVÖLGYI et al. 1979).

3.3 Xeroradiography

Xeroradiography is a technique specifically geared towards the examination of soft tissue. The theoretical background and applicability of
xeroradiography has been worked out in several papers (OLIPHANT 1955;
ROACH and HILLEBOE 1955 a, b; BOAG 1973; WOLFE 1973). It combines the
use of less penetrating, soft X-rays with, instead of X-ray film, an aluminum
plate coated with a positively charged layer of selenium which is exposed as
a normal X-ray plate. The X-rays pass through the soft tissue and strike the
positively charged selenium layer, thereby discharging it and producing
positive and negative charges in proportion to the characteristics of the penetrating X-rays. A cloud of negatively charged ink powder is then sprayed
into the developing chamber, producing a pattern induced by the charged
selenium. The powder is then transferred to paper by an electrostatic process and fixed by heat. The technique gives a weak overall contrast but a
sharp and characteristic intensity of borders.

Xeroradiography has been shown to be clinically effective in many applications such as mammography (LUTTERBECK 1972; WOLFE 1972), examination of axillary lymph nodes (KALISHER 1975), juxtaosseous soft tissues
(WOLFE 1969; OTTO et al. 1976) and the tracheobronchial tree (DOUST and
TING 1974; HARLE et al. 1975; JING 1974).

The use of xeroradiography for the study of the normal and pathological muscular system has so far been relatively limited. In a first publication
PÁLVÖLGYI and PÉNTEK (1977) presented a series of xerograms of the normal musculature of arms and legs. The same year a small study of 30 patients was published, in which xeroradiographic and normal soft tissue
radiograms were compared (PÁLVÖLGY et al. 1977). They found that
xeroradiography of muscles gave more harmonious pictures with a better
outline of the fatty degenerations, muscle contours, calcifications and oede-
mas. Despite the rather limited use of this technique in the examination of
muscles the possibilities of xeroradiography are obvious (Figs. 3.3, and
3.4), and a comprehensive study on a large series of various pathologies is
certainly indicated. According to OSTERMAN et al. (1977), the quality of the
images can be further enhanced by using negative-mode imaging.

3.4 Radioisotope Uptake in Skeletal Muscle

Radioisotope techniques have been used for many years to study the
composition of the human body and the sizes of its different compartments
(BROZEK 1963). Body potassium is an especially interesting parameter for
studying the skeletal muscular compartment because of its selective associ-

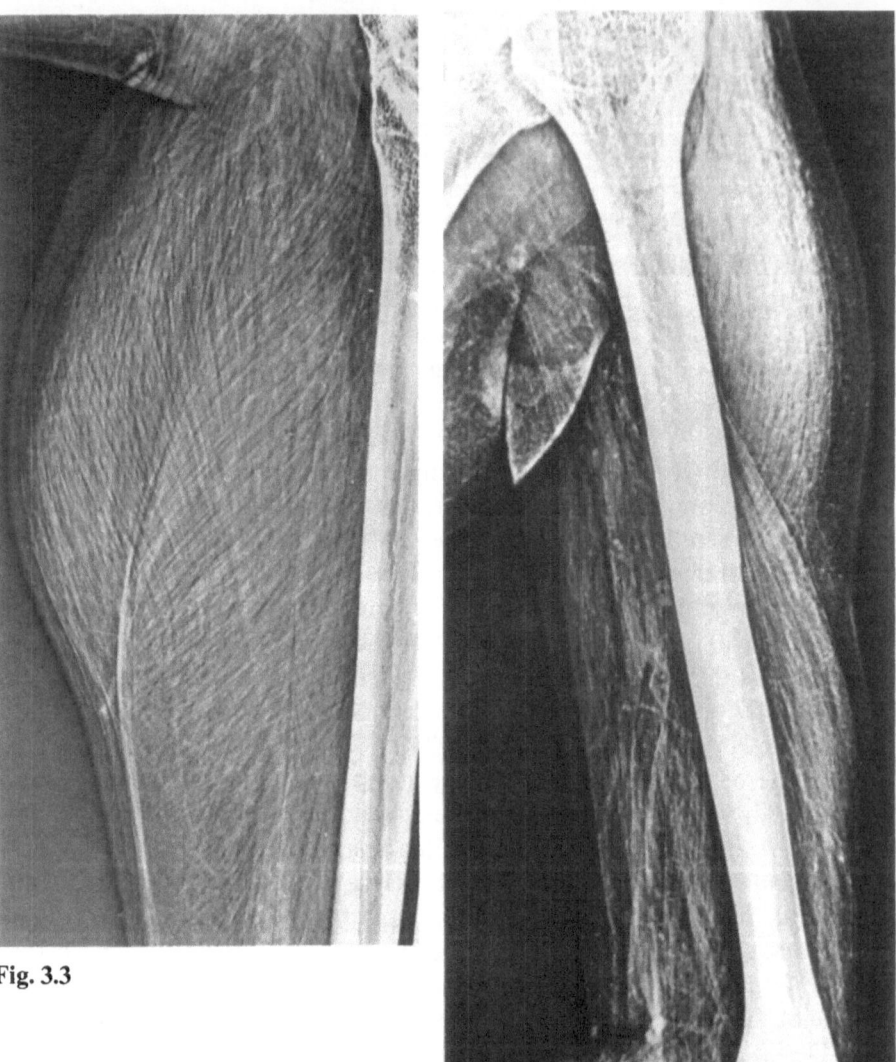

Fig. 3.3

Fig. 3.4

Fig. 3.3. Lateral xeroradiogram of the calf muscles of a patient with pseudo-hypertrophic muscular dystrophy. Fine striation is seen in the m. triceps surae, which is otherwise well preserved. (Courtesy of R. PÁLVÖLGYI, M. D., Priv. Doz.)

Fig. 3.4. Lateral xeroradiogram of the upper arm muscles of a patient with progressive muscular dystrophy. The m. biceps brachii is severely affected. Moderate muscular destruction of the fibres of the m. triceps brachii is observed, while m. deltoideus shows only fine striation. (Courtesy of R. PÁLVÖLGYI, M. D., Priv. Doz.)

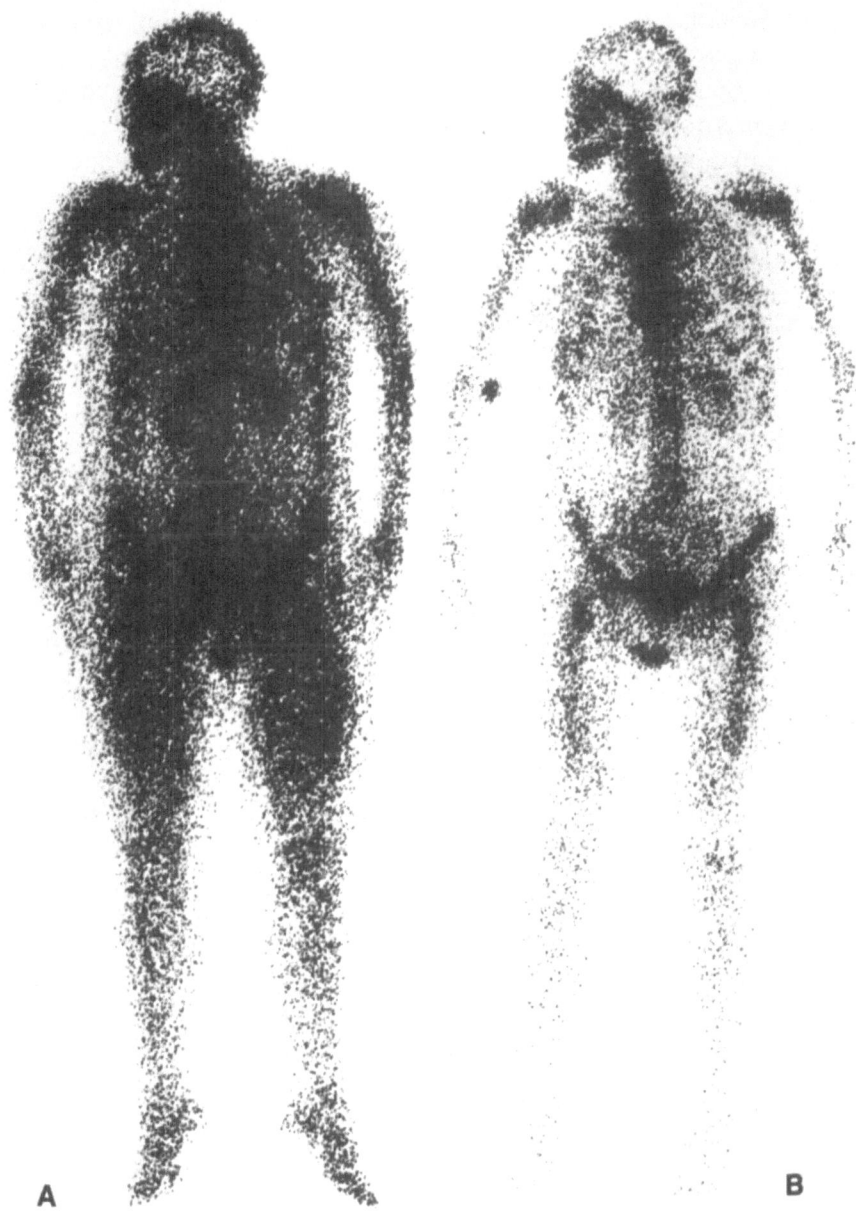

Fig. 3.5 A, B. Radio-isotope scanning, with ^{99m}Tc-pyrophosphate, of a 41-year- old female with subacute polymyositis. In **A** the patient is shown at the onset of the disease. The radioisotope uptake in muscle exceeds that in bone. In **B** the same patient is shown after 6 months of high-dose prednisone treatment. All biochemical parameters have returned to normal, including serum CK. The muscular radioisotope uptake has returned to normal as well

ation with the proteins of the muscle mass. Of total body potassium, 95% is intracellular, a large part being intramuscular as well. BLAHD et al. (1967) and KOSSMANN et al. (1965) described marked decreases in total body potassium in cases of muscular atrophy of various kinds. DELWAIDE et al. (1972) demonstrated a lowered body potassium in three types of neuromuscular disease: muscular dystrophy, neurogenic amyotrophy and myasthenia gravis.

Much more specific and useful, however, is the use of ^{99m}Tc-pyrophosphate. RUSSELL et al. (1969, 1970) have demonstrated that pyrophosphate is a physiological regulator of calcium and phosphate metabolism in bone. BUYA et al. (1975) studied morphological correlates of ^{99m}Tc-stannous pyrophosphate imaging of acute heart muscle infarcts in dogs. They concluded that there was a correlation of temporal changes in the scintigraphic findings and in the content of demonstrable calcium deposits in infarcts, and a correlation between sites of localization of calcified muscle cells and high radioactivity levels in the lesions.

Calcification of muscle due to the deposition of amorphous calcium in the absence of osteoblastic activity seems to be one of the major consequences of muscle cell necrosis. KARPATI (1977) and SCHOTLAND et al. (1979) have demonstrated the focal defects in the muscle cell surface membrane may be the earliest morphological abnormality in Duchenne muscular dystrophy. This structural defect would permit the outflow of muscle enzymes such as creatine kinase but also the inflow of calcium-rich extracellular fluid into the cell. Mitochondria accumulate this excess calcium, and the calcium overload in turn is responsible for decreased ATP formation, which is critical for calcium pumps in the sarcoplasmic reticulum and plasma membrane. When calcium concentration exceeds critical levels protein synthesis stalls, hypercontraction is activated and calcium-sensitive proteases are activated; this eventually leads to cell necrosis (BUSCH et al. 1972; MOKRI and ENGEL 1975; WROGEMAN and PENA 1976; W. K. ENGEL 1977; BODENSTEINER and ENGEL 1978; DUNCAN 1978).

When large areas of muscular necrosis accumulate calcium, they can be demonstrated by ^{99m}Tc-methylene diphosphonate or ^{99m}Tc-pyrophosphate (Fig. 3.5). This has been extensively proven (SUZUKI et al. 1974; SARMIENTO et al. 1975; SIEGEL et al. 1975; SPIES et al. 1975; KRISHNAMURTHY et al. 1975; STEINFELD et al. 1976; BROWN et al. 1976; BELLINA et al. 1978; SWIFT and BROWN 1978; SILBERSTEIN and BOVE 1979; DESAI et al. 1980; VITA and HARRIS 1981; BRILL 1981).

SIEGEL et al. (1975) and W. K. ENGEL (1977) have demonstrated that ^{99m}Tc-diphosphonate accumulation in muscles damaged by experimentally induced ischaemia correlated with calcium accumulation, and that this was directly proportional to circulating CK levels and loss of potassium from damaged muscles.

4 Computed Tomography Applied to the Human Skeletal Muscular System

It is beyond the scope of this work to describe in detail technical data about scanning and image processing with the different scanner types used. Nevertheless, some practical information concerning the scanning instruments and methods, the densitometric readings and the photographic reproduction is necessary for a good understanding of the images.

4.1 Scanning Instruments

Three different types of CT scanners were used to examine the patients' muscular systems: the Δ 50 (Ohio Nuclear Co.), the Somatom 2 (Siemens) and the Δ 2020 (Ohio Nuclear Co.). The main characteristics of the instruments and the scanning parameters used are summarized in Table 4.1. The Δ 50 scanner produces two simultaneous slices of 13 mm thickness with a translation-rotation movement. The number of detectors is three per slice produced, i.e. six. The scan time varies between 120 and 150 s, depending upon the chosen scan diameter (20–45 cm). To improve spatial resolution the smallest possible scan diameter was always selected, the pixel surface varying, on the 256×256 matrix, from 0.6 mm² on a 20-cm scan diameter to almost 3 mm² on a 45-cm scan diameter. Image display is produced with window settings of 640 and a centre of 30 on the classical Hounsfield scale.

The working of the Somatom 2 CT scanner is based on the rotatory detector (fan beam) principle with 512 detectors ranged in a curve of 42° in front of the X-ray tube. The image is realized by a complete rotation over 360° of both X-ray tube and detectors. The Somatom 2 is able to produce 2-, 4- or 8-mm slices. Scan time can be chosen as either 3,5 or 10 s. The scan diameter can vary between 25 and 45 cm with a pixel surface of 1–3 mm².

The "zoom factor" software program allows an enlargement of the image, with improvement of the spatial resolution. The matrix is of 256×256 points. Average settings on Somatom 2 for standard muscle examination are given in Table 4.2. Window settings used on Somatom 2 are 512 with a centre of 30.

Table 4.1. Main characteristics of instruments and scanning parameters of the different scanners used

	Δ 50	Somatom 2	Δ 2020
Movement X-ray tube and detector group	Translation-rotation	Rotatory detector (fan beam)	Stationary detector
Scan time	120 – 150 s (for 2 contiguous scans)[a]	3, 5, 10 s	2, 4, 8, 16 s
Slice thickness	13 mm	2, 4, 8 mm	4, 7, 10 mm
Image matrix	256 × 256 pts	256 × 256 pts	512 × 512 pts
Milliamperes/per second	30 × 120 à 150	460 – 230	50, 75 – 150
Kilovolts	125	120	120
Diameter	20, 35, 45 cm	25 – 45 cm	25, 40, 50 cm

[a] Scan time depending on object diameter: 20 – 45 cm

Table 4.2. Settings for Somatom 2 scanner for standard skeletal muscle examination

Tilt	mA/s	kV	SLT (mm)	ST (s)	WIND	CE	DIA
0	460	120	2	3	512	30	Maximal enlargement

SLT, slice thickness; ST, scan time; WIND, window setting; CE, centre; DIA, diameter

Table 4.3. Settings for Δ 2020 scanner for standard skeletal muscle examination

	Level 1	Level 2	Level 3	Level 4	Level 5
Tilt	− 3° to + 3°	0	0	0	0
mA/s	50.0	75.0	75.0	75.0	75.0
kV	120.0	120.0	120.0	120.0	120.0
CFF	1	1	1	1	1
SLT (mm)	10.0	7.0	7.0	7.0	7.0
ST (s)	2	2	2	2	2
WIND	640	640	640	640	640
CE	30	30	30	30	30
DIA (cm)	25	40/50	40/50	40/50	40/50

CFF, convolver filter function; SLT, slice thickness; ST, scan time; WIND, window setting; CE, centre; DIA, diameter

The $\varDelta$ 2020 CT scanner is a stationary detector scanner with 720 detectors ranged at the outside of the tube trajectory. The tube performs a complete rotation in 2, 4 or 8 s.

Scan diameter varies between 25, 40 and 50 cm, with a pixel surface varying between 0.25, 0.6 and 1 mm² on the matrix of 512×512 points; the thickness varies between 4, 7 and 10 mm. Average table settings for the $\varDelta$ 2020 for standard muscle examination are shown in Table 4.3. Window settings chosen on $\varDelta$ 2020 are of 600 with a centre of 30.

The surface dose for the three different instruments varies from 0.7 to 1.5 mGy per slice (MacCullough et al. 1978; Trefler and Haughton 1981).

4.2 Densitometric Readings

Numerical densitometry in CT provides information about the specific gravity of the tissue examined. Image display controls and numerical output data are expressed in Hounsfield Units (HU). The HU expresses the attenuation value at a matrix point relative to the attenuation value for water calculated as follows: $HU_{xy} = 1000 \cdot (\mu_{xy} - \mu_w) \cdot \mu_w^{-1}$, where μ_w represents the average attenuation value of water and μ_{xy} the average attenuation value at a given matrix location xy (Ter-Pogossian 1977).

From a practical point of view, the measurement of density is performed by adjusting and determining a region of interest, from which size and shape can be adapted. Mean density of the chosen region of interest, number of matrix points (pixels), calculated area and various statistical values are displayed.

Only with the $\varDelta$ 50 is the standard deviation of the mean reported by the computer with each measurement. These standard deviations of the mean Hounsfield numbers were found to be uniformly small in all normal cases.

Some programs allow the display of the densitometric values in a chosen area as a histogram illustrating the density value dispersion in the area. This variance is at the base of the densitometric error if the region of interest is too small. The minimum surface of the region of interest which allows reliable densitometry is 20 pixels with the $\varDelta$ 50, the Somatom and the $\varDelta$ 2020, covering a different surface of course, according to the instrument and the diameter chosen.

Limitations and errors of densitometry are mainly due to densitometric pollution and partial volume averaging.

The first general aspect of absolute numerical densitometry to be remembered is its dependence upon apparatus characteristics. Spectral shift

error, non-linearity, image noise and resistance to high- or low-density artefacts are fundamental problems not solved equally well in all equipment
(BELLON et al. 1979; HOUNSFIELD 1976; HOUNSFIELD 1978; LATCHAW et al.
1977; MACCULLOUGH 1977). The complexity of these problems is ac-
centuated by the great variability of the subjects to be examined: patients'
shape, habitus and centering are all factors influencing the final results.

Densitometric pollution can arise from basic meteorological or radiological changes, the ground noise and the artefacts. The most aberrant densities are measured at the transition area between high- and low-density.
Image degradation and densitometric pollution of high-density material,
such as osteosynthesis material or barium rest, do not require any com-
ment.

Partial volume averaging concerns structures that do not fill the entire
slice thickness. It originates from the mixture of densities of different structures coexisting in a slice thickness and will lead to erroneous densitometry awing to the averaging of the density of the lesion or area to be
measured with that of the adjoining areas in the same slice thickness. The
importance of this partial volume averaging decreases, of course, with the
use of very small slice thicknesses.

The mean densitometric values of normal muscular tissue on the HU
scale vary between 30 and 80 HU, depending mainly upon the muscle
group measured (BULCKE et al. 1979a, MATEGRANO et al. 1977).

4.3 Photography

For video monitoring or for photographic documentation in our investigations, each matrix point in the display was modulated for intensity or
colour in accordance with the corresponding HU. Hence, the display represents a map of the linear attenuation coefficients within the area scanned.
The display gain (grey scale or colour spectrum from minimum to maximum) and offset could be adjusted to encompass a display window over the
HU range of interest. This allowed a selected small range of HU values to
be displayed over the entire video spectrum. HU values above the upper
window limit were displayed at maximum scale and HU values below the
lower window limit were displayed at minimum scale. HU values between
the upper and lower limits were displayed in accordance with the calibra-
tion stripe. So, for a good interpretation of a section through the thigh
muscles, it was necessary to visualize the skin, the panniculus adiposus, the
fatty infiltration of the muscle bundles and the bony structures, with their
respective alteration. A 500 window was therefore required because of the
large difference in X-ray absorption of the displayed tissues. For video

monitoring and routine image reproduction for clinical interpretative use, the 'positive' display and printing method was used, the images being viewed or reproduced on a black background. For routine clinical study the images were reproduced on transparent X-ray film with a 70 mm camera (Hasselblad) or a multiformat camera (Matrix, Deltamat). Otherwise, images are stored on floppy disks or magnetic tapes in order to allow further densitometric or window study of the material.

Photographic reproduction in this book was filmed from the monitor for some images or reproduced from the multiformat images. For the photographic reproduction, negative printing was chosen, based on the subjective idea that minimal differences in density are better visible in the clear area of the grey-scale spectrum. This appeared of great value in severe muscle atrophy, where on the positive images the rare spared muscles were lost in the dark of the surrounding fat.

For a good understanding of the reproduced images it is essential to consider that we photographed the right side of the patient, which is on the left side of the picture according to international convention.

5 A Standard Procedure for Examination of the Human Skeletal Muscular System

5.1 Why a Standard Examination Procedure?

The human skeletal muscular system consists of a large number of striated muscles with a wide variation in size and functional significance, from the very small mm. bulbi and m. stapedius to the large m. quadriceps. In principle all these muscles can be visualized by CT scanning. In clinical practice, however, for which the present procedure is intended, the dose of radiation and the time required for such examinations are prohibitive, the precise identification of many muscles remains difficult and the diagnostic and therapeutic value of the description of lesions in an individual muscle is often rather irrelevant. Limiting the CT examination to a number of well-selected scan levels thus seemed a mandatory requirement for making it acceptable as a routine procedure in the examination of myopathies.

The selection of standard CT scan levels was guided by a few well-defined objectives. First, the clinical experience that in many myopathies certain muscle groups are affected more frequently and earlier than others was taken into account. Next, regions were chosen where the ratio of the number and total area of muscular shadows to areas of osseous and other structures was found to be maximal. Finally, several levels had to be excluded as unsuitable for routine examination because radiological artefacts were almost always present. This was particularly the case with the forearm muscles. Probably due to the high bone-soft tissue ratio in this area, the CT images remained unsatisfactory despite many technical attempts to eliminate them. Fortunately however, muscular lesions of the forearm, in contrast to those of the limb-girdle muscles, are more easily approachable by clinical means, which makes CT scanning of the arms less useful.

As in every other radiological examination, CT scans of the pathological skeletal muscular system can only be interpreted by comparing them with normal CT scans, and this comparison is only meaningful when the pathological scans are as closely congruent as possible with the normal ones. To make this possible, each of the standard levels has to be well defined by easily recognizable superficial focusing points which can first be marked on

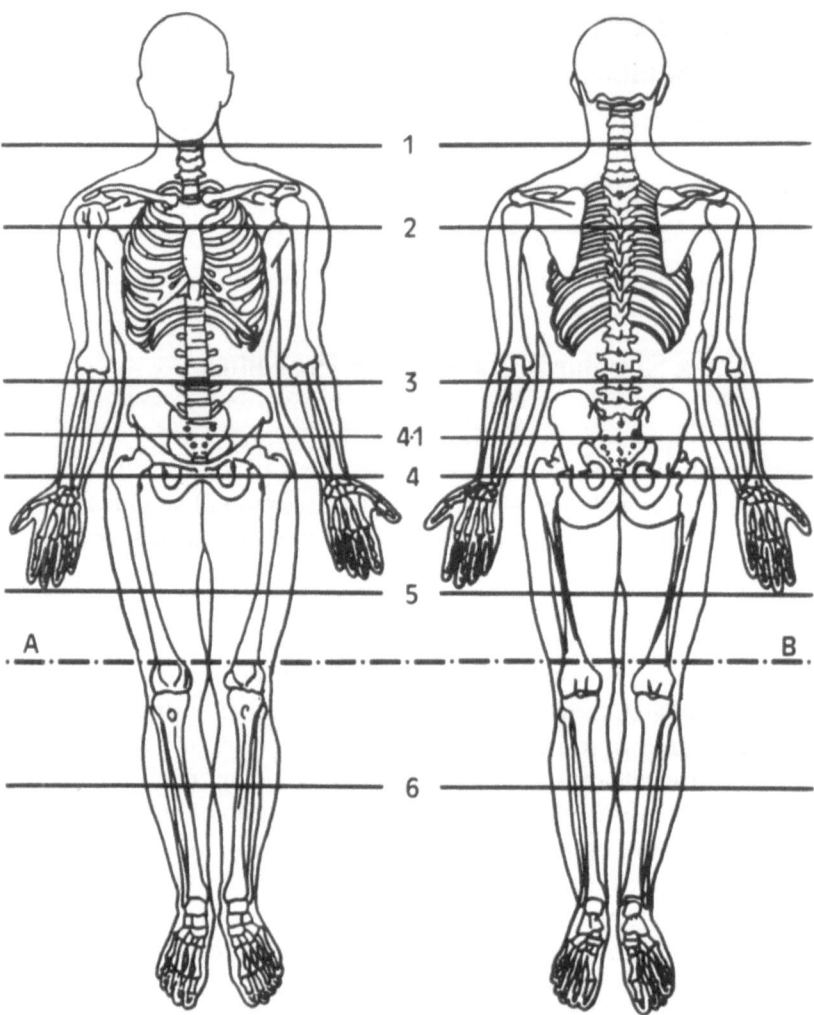

Fig. 5.1. Levels scanned in the standard examination procedure. *1*, the neck muscles; *2*, the shoulder girdle muscles; *3*, the abdominal wall and spinal muscles; *4*, the pelvic muscles; *5*, the thigh muscles; *6*, the lower leg muscles. The *line 4.1* represents the focus of our early scanning procedures through the middle of the ligamentum inguinale. Scans through this line are very suitable for demonstrating the mm. glutei complex as shown in Figs. 5.12 and 5.13. It is the only scan which differs significantly from the standard examination procedure. Several pathological scans shown in the text were also taken through this focus. The *dotted line A–B* runs through the upper edges of both patellae, and serves as reference for *lines 5* and *6*. How these lines were defined for the different scanners is described in Table 5.1

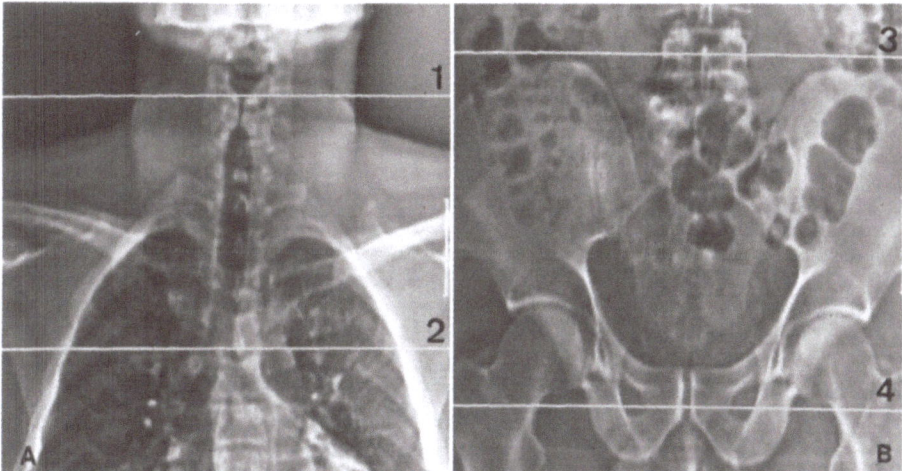

Fig. 5.2 A, B. Radiological focusing lines of **A** levels 1 and 2 and **B** levels 3 and 4 as they can be visualized on late-model scanners on topographic displays prior to scanning. This is particularly useful in obese patients when external markers are difficult to localize

the skin; the scanner can then be focused on them by means of built-in localizer light beams. With the Somatom 2 scanner preliminary topographic X-rays of the area to be examined were obtained on the video monitor, on which the focusing points could then be plotted with great accuracy. This was sometimes found to be particularly useful in obese patients. In the majority of cases the radiological pictures obtained through these focusing points were well standardized, but even then variation was possible. Therefore during the examination the scan level was sometimes corrected, based on purely radiological markers.

Six transverse scans at six different levels of the body were finally selected which, combined, form the standard examination procedure used throughout this book. They are (1) the neck muscles, (2) the shoulder muscles, (3) the abdominal wall and spinal muscles, (4) the pelvic muscles, (5) the thigh muscles and (6) the lower leg muscles. As we have successively worked with three different scanning instruments, a Δ 50, a Δ 2020 and a Somatom 2 scanner, the standard levels chosen, the definition of their focusing points and radiological markers have undergone some changes which are summarized in Table 5.1 and Fig. 5.1. A description of these changes was felt to be necessary in order to understand the variation which will be observed when, for example, follow-up pictures are presented. The general appearance of the scans, however, has not substantially changed with the different scanners. Therefore in this chapter we have presented standard pictures made with our most recent scanner as representative for

Table 5.1. Scanning levels, superficial focusing points and radiological characteristics of the standard examination procedure

Level	Δ50		Δ2020		Somatom 2	
	Focusing point	Radiological characteristics	Focusing point	Radiological characteristics	Focusing point	Radiological characteristics
1 Neck muscles	Upper edge of cartilago thyroidea	a	Prominentia laryngea of cartilago thyroidea	Sharp triangular shape of cartilago thyroidea	Prominentia laryngea of cartilago thyroidea	Sharp triangular shape of cartilago thyroidea
2 Shoulder muscles	Largest diameter of upper arm (through m. deltoideus)	a	Manubrium sterni	Elongated linear aspect of the scapula	Manubrium sterni	Elongated linear aspect of the scapula
3 Abdominal wall and spinal muscles	b	a, b	a, b	a	1 cm above upper edges of cristae iliacae	Largest shadow of m. psoas major
4 Pelvic muscles	Middle of ligamentum inguinale	a	Middle of symphysis pubica	Maximum distance between symphysis pubica, os femoris and os ischii	Middle of symphysis pubica	Maximum distance between symphysis pubica, os femoris and os ischii
5 Thigh muscles	Largest diameter of thigh	a	15 cm above upper edge of patella	Os femoris	15 cm above upper edge of patella	Os femoris
6 Lower leg muscles	Largest diameter of lower leg	a	20 cm below upper edge of patella	Tibia and fibula	20 cm below upper edge of patella	Tibia and fibula

a In the Δ50 examinations no re-adjustments of scan levels on the basis of radiological characteristics were allowed
b Not carried out in this examination

the standard procedure. The radiological levels of these scans are shown in Fig. 5.2.

The maximum number of muscles which can be seen within the normal variability of the standard examination procedure is about 70 on each side of the body. This is a sizeable sample of the total number of skeletal muscles and also represents a wide range of motor nerves and motor neuron pools. The standard examination procedure is therefore a suitable instrument for the investigation not only of myopathies but also of peripheral neuropathies and medullary lesions.

5.2 Radiological and Anatomical Description of the Normal Human Skeletal Muscular System by the Standard Examination Procedure

We will now entensively describe the normal appearance at each of the six levels of the standard examination procedure. On each level striated muscles belonging to different anatomical and functional groups are seen. Therefore each scan description is preceded by one or several tables describing these groups of muscles within their functional context, together with their motor nerves, the spinal segment levels of their motor neuron pools and their main actions. These tables should be useful for a better understanding of the relationship between the questions asked and the information given by the clinician and radiological findings.

Most classical anatomical textbooks follow subdivision schemes very similar to the ones described in these tables, but one exception needs to be discussed. In the *Nomina Anatomica* (WARWICK 1977) which we have used throughout this text, and which is used in most classical textbooks, the m. extensor spinae is only one of many extensor muscles of the spine (musculi dorsi, mm. dorsi). In some anatomy and kinesiology textbooks, however, m. extensor spinae is employed as synonymous with mm. dorsi, and all other muscles of the back are classified under its heading (SCHADÉ 1974; RASH and BURKE 1978). We have followed this trend in previous papers (BULCKE et al. 1979a; TERMOTE et al. 1980), but in the present text we return to the classical definition as described in Table 5.6.

As will be seen in the following figures, one of the main features of the normal skeletal muscular system is the dense packing of the different muscles, which sometimes makes the anatomical description of individual muscles rather difficult. The muscular anatomy in vivo as seen by CT scan is certainly different from the anatomy described on anatomical preparations from which the normal tissue consistency has disappeared. This may be the major reason why some textbooks on total-body CT scanning

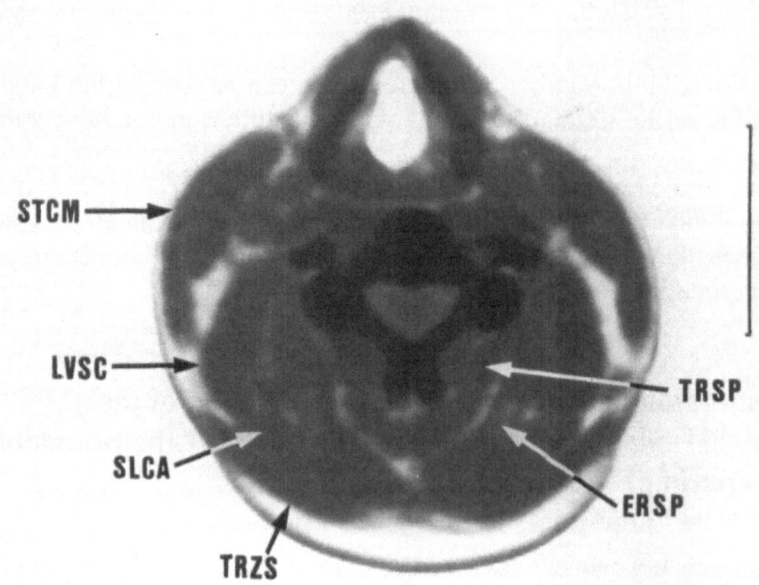

Fig. 5.3. Standard CT scan of the normal neck musculature. Linear magnification compared with shoulder muscles in Fig. 5.5, approximately 2.2 times. The separation between the m. transversospinalis (*TRSP*) and m. erector spinae (*ERSP*) is almost always clearly visible. Further landmarks at this level are the m. sternocleidomastoideus (*STCM*), m. levator scapulae (*LVSC*), m. splenius capitis (*SLCA*) and m. trapezius (*TRZS*). Bar = 5 cm

have given so little attention to the skeletal muscular system. GAMBARELLI et al. (1977) provide excellent drawings of their CT scans on which all muscles are very clearly outlined, but in only a few pictures can the names of the muscles be found. The same is true for ALFIDI et al. (1977). In LED-LEY et al. (1977) and MESCHAN (1978), however, all muscles are clearly marked. When in doubt, we have therefore turned to the latter texts for advice on muscular anatomy.

5.2.1 The Neck Muscle Level

The first CT scan of the standard examination procedure consists of a transverse section through the neck at the level of the cartilago thyroidea. The standard picture is taken with the patient in the supine position. The focusing points are described in Table 5.1 and in Figs. 5.1 and 5.2. During the scanning the patient is asked not to move, breathe or swallow.

In Fig. 5.3 a standard neck muscle scan is shown. The main radiological characteristic of this level is the sharp triangular shape of the cartilago thyroidea with its forward-projecting edge. The vertebral body appearing in

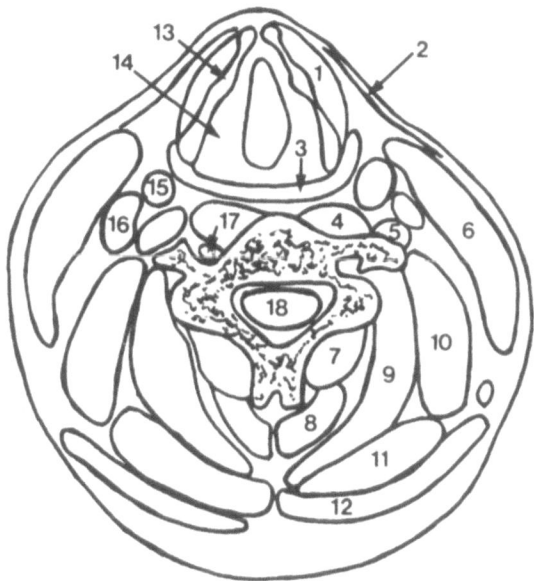

Fig. 5.4. Line drawing of the CT scan shown in Fig. 5.3. *1,* mm. infrahyoidei: m. thyrohyoideus, m. sternohyoideus, m. omohyoideus; *2,* platysma; *3,* m. constrictor pharyngis inferior; *4,* m. longus colli; *5,* m. scalenus anterior; *6,* m. sternocleidomastoideus; *7,* m. multifidus; *8,* m. semispinalis capitis; *9,* m. longissimus cervicis, m. splenius cervicis; *10,* m. levator scapulae; *11,* m. splenius capitis; *12,* m. trapezius; *13,* cartilago thyroidea; 14, plica vestibularis; *15,* arteria carotis communis (near bifurcation); *16,* vena jugularis interna; *17, (arrow)* arteria vertebralis; *18,* medulla spinalis

the scan is C4. As can be seen, the neck level contains a large number of muscles which belong to several anatomical groups (Tables 5.2–5.6). The extensor muscles of the spine (mm. dorsi), summarized in Table 5.6, have been included here because they do start in the neck, although they are perhaps better developed at lower levels. Anteriorly in the scan we find the intricate structures of the pharynx and the larynx. The changes in some of these muscles have been subjected to very detailed CT examinations during phonation and quiet breathing (GAMSU et al. 1981), and although these changes will be observed in our scans, they certainly exceed the scope of this work and will not be commented upon.

What is usually clearly visible in this cross section is the separation between – as described in Table 5.6 (mm. dorsi) – the deep oblique back muscles, represented by the m. transversospinalis and the long straight muscles represented by the m. erector spinae. The distinctions between the three layers of the former and the three columns of the latter (ANDERSON 1978) are, however, barely visible at this level. In previous papers (BULCKE et al. 1979 a; TERMOTE et al. 1980) we described the m. transversospinalis as mm. erectores spinae, for reasons already explained, while the long straight

Table 5.2. Striated larynx muscles (musculi laryngis)

	Muscle	Motor nerve	Motor neuron pool	Action
1	*External muscles*			
1.1	m. thyrohyoideus	Ansa cervicalis [n. hypoglossus (XII)]	C1-C3	Elevation of cartilago thyroidea / Depression of os hyoideum
1.2	m. mylohyoideus	n. trigeminus (V), n. mylohyoideus	Motor nu. n. trigemini	Elevation of os hyoideum and tongue
1.3	m. geniohyoideus	Ansa cervicalis [n. hypoglossus (XII)]	C1-C3	Forward movement of os hyoideum and tongue
1.4	m. digastricus venter posterior	n. facialis (VII), r. digastricus	Motor nu. n. facialis	Elevation of os hyoideum
	venter anterior	n. trigeminus (V), n. mylohyoideus	Motor nu. n. trigemini	Assistance opening jaws / Elevation and retraction of os hyoideum and tongue
1.5	m. palatopharyngeus	Plexus pharyngeus [n. glossopharyngeus (IX) and n. vagus (X)]	nu. ambiguus	Elevation of pharynx / Assistance closing nasopharynx
1.6	m. constrictor pharyngis inferior	n. vagus (X), n. laryngeus superior	nu. ambiguus	Contraction of lower pharynx
2	*Internal muscles*			
2.1	m. cricothyroideus	n. vagus (X), n. laryngeus superior, r. externus	nu. ambiguus	Produces tension and elongation of vocal cords
2.2	m. cricoarytenoideus posterior	n. vagus (X), n. laryngeus superior	nu. ambiguus	Opens glottis by rotating cartilago arytenoidea outwards
2.3	m. cricoarytenoideus lateralis	n. vagus (X), n. laryngeus superior	nu. ambiguus	Closes glottis by rotating cartilago arytenoidea inwards
2.4	m. arytenoideus transversus	n. vagus (X), n. laryngeus superior	nu. ambiguus	Closes glottis opening by pulling cartilagines arytenoidae together
2.5	m. arytenoideus obliquus	n. vagus (X), n. laryngeus superior	nu. ambiguus	Closes glottis opening by pulling cartilagines arytenoidae together
2.6	m. aryepiglotticus	n. vagus (X), n. laryngeus superior	nu. ambiguus	Closes glottis opening by pulling cartilagines arytenoidae together
2.7	m. thyroepiglotticus	n. vagus (X), n. laryngeus superior	nu. ambiguus	Brings vocal cords together

Table 5.3. Striated pharynx muscles (tunica muscularis pharyngis)

	Muscle	Motor nerve	Motor neuron pool	Action
1	*Circular muscles*			
1.1	m. constrictor pharyngis superior	Plexus pharyngeus [n. glosso-pharyngeus (IX) and n. vagus (X)]	nu. ambiguus	Contraction of upper pharynx
1.2	m. constrictor pharyngis medius	Plexus pharyngeus [n. glosso-pharyngeus (IX) and n. vagus (X)]	nu. ambiguus	Contraction of middle pharynx
1.3	m. constrictor pharyngis inferior	n. vagus (X), n. laryngeus superior	nu. ambiguus	Contraction of lower pharynx
2	*Longitudinal muscles*			
2.1	m. stylopharyngeus	n. glossopharyngeus (IX), r. m. stylopharyngei	nu. ambiguus	Elevates and dilates pharynx
2.2	m. palatopharyngeus	Plexus pharyngeus [n. glosso-pharyngeus (IX) and n. vagus (X)]	nu. ambiguus	Elevates pharynx. Assists closing nasopharynx

Table 5.4. Cervico-occipital muscles (musculi capitis)

	Muscle	Motor nerve	Motor neuron pool	Action
1	m. rectus capitis posterior major	n. suboccipitalis	C1	Extension and rotation of head
2	m. rectus capitis posterior minor	n. suboccipitalis	C1	Extension and rotation of head
3	m. rectus capitis lateralis	n. suboccipitalis	C1	Lateral flexion of head
4	m. obliquus capitis superior	n. suboccipitalis	C1	Extension and lateral flexion of head
5	m. obliquus capitis inferior	n. suboccipitalis	C1 or C2	Rotation of atlas

Table 5.5. Neck muscles (musculi colli)

	Muscle	Motor nerve	Motor neuron pool	Action
1	*Superficial layer*			
1.1	Platysma	n. facialis (VII)	Motor nu. n. facialis	Depression of mandibula Depression of lower lip Wrinkling of skin of neck
1.2	m. sternocleidomastoideus	n. accessorius (XI) and branches of plexus cervicalis	nu. ambiguus C2-C3	Bending of head and neck towards shoulder; Rotation of head towards opposite side; Raising of sternum (head fixed); Inspiration
2	*Middle layer*			
2.1	mm. infrahyoidei	Ansa cervicalis [n. hypoglossus (XII)]	C1-C3	Downward movement of os hyoideum
2.2	m. sternohyoideus	Ansa cervicalis [n. hypoglossus (XII)]	C1-C3	Downward movement of os hyoideum
2.3	m. omohyoideus	Ansa cervicalis [n. hypoglossus (XII)]	C1-C3	Depression of cartilago thyroidea
2.4	m. sternothyroideus	Ansa cervicalis [n. hypoglossus (XII)]	C1-C2	Elevation of cartilago thyroidea
2.5	m. thyrohyoideus	Ansa cervicalis [n. hypoglossus (XII)]	C1-C3	Depression of os hyoideum
2.6	m. levator glandulae thyroideae			
3	*Deep layer*			
3.1	*Lateral deep layer*			
3.1.1	m. scalenus anterior	Branches of plexus cervicalis and of plexus brachialis	C5-C7	Elevation of rib 1 Flexion and slight rotation of neck Inspiration

3.1.2	m. scalenus medius	Branches of plexus cervicalis and of plexus brachialis	C2-C8	Elevation of rib 1 Flexion and slight rotation of neck Inspiration
3.1.3	m. scalenus posterior	Branches of plexus cervicalis and of plexus brachialis	C5-C8	Elevation of rib 2 Flexion and slight rotation of neck Inspiration
3.2	*Prevertebral muscles*			
3.2.1	m. longus colli	Branches of plexus cervicalis	C1-C5	Flexion of neck Slight rotation of cervical spine
3.2.2	m. longus capitis	Branches of plexus cervicalis	C1-C4	Rotation of head (unilateral action) Bending head forward (bilateral action)
3.2.3	m. rectus capitis anterior	n. suboccipitalis	C1	Bending of head and shoulder (unilateral action) Bending head forward (bilateral action)

Table 5.6. Extensor muscles of the spine (musculi dorsi)

	Muscle	Motor nerve	Motor neu-ron pool	Action
1	*Spinocostalis*			
1.1	m. serratus posterior superior	nn. intercostales	T1-T4	Elevation of ribs Enlargement of thorax
1.2	m. serratus posterior inferior	nn. intercostales	T9-T12	Drawing downward and backward of lower four ribs
2	*Spinotransversarius*			
2.1	m. splenius	dorsal branches from cervical spinal cord	C2-C5 (C6)	Extension and rotation of neck
2.1.1	m. splenius cervicis	dorsal branches from cervical spinal cord	C2-C5 (C6)	Flexion of neck to side
2.1.2	m. splenius capitis	dorsal branches from cervical spinal cord	C2-C5 (C6)	Extension and rotation of neck Flexion of neck to side
3	*Long straight muscles*			
3.1	*m. erector spinae*			
3.1.1	*m. iliocostalis*	rr. dorsales from nn. spinales	C1-L5	
3.1.1.1	m. iliocostalis lumborum	rr. dorsales from nn. spinales		Extension of thoracic spine
3.1.1.2	m. iliocostalis thoracis	rr. dorsales from nn. spinales		Extension of cervical spine
3.1.1.3	m. iliocostalis cervicis	rr. dorsales from nn. spinales		Extension of cervical spine
3.1.2	*m. longissimus*	rr. dorsales from nn. spinales	C1-L5	
3.1.2.1	m. longissimus thoracis	rr. dorsales from nn. spinales		Extension of thoracic spine Flexion of thoracic spine to one side Draws ribs downward

3.1.2.2	m. longissimus cervicis	rr. dorsales from nn. spinales	Extension of cervical spine Flexion of cervical spine to one side
3.1.2.3	m. longissimus capitis	rr. dorsales from nn. spinales	Extension of head Flexion of head to one side Slight rotation of head
3.1.3	*m. spinalis*	rr. dorsales from nn. spinales	C2–L1
3.1.3.1	m. spinalis thoracis	rr. dorsales from nn. spinales	Extension of thoracic spine
3.1.3.2	m. spinalis cervicis	rr. dorsales from nn. spinales	Extension of cervical spine
3.1.3.3	m. spinalis capitis	rr. dorsales from nn. spinales	Extension of head
4	*Oblique back muscles*		
4	*m. transversospinalis*		
4.1	*m. semispinalis*	rr. dorsales from nn. spinales	C1–T6
4.1.1	m. semispinalis thoracis	rr. dorsales from nn. spinales	Extension and rotation of spine
4.1.2	m. semispinalis cervicis	rr. dorsales from nn. spinales	Extension and rotation of spine
4.1.3	m. semispinalis capitis	rr. dorsales from nn. spinales	Extension and rotation of head
4.2	*m. multifidus*	rr. dorsales from nn. spinales	C3–S3
4.3	*mm. rotatores*	rr. dorsales from nn. spinales	C1–L5
4.3.1	mm. rotatores lumborum	rr. dorsales from nn. spinales	Extension and rotation of spine
4.3.2	mm. rotatores thoracis	rr. dorsales from nn. spinales	Extension and rotation of spine
4.3.3	mm. rotatores cervicis	rr. dorsales from nn. spinales	Extension and rotation of spine
5	*Short straight muscles*		
5.1	*mm. intertransversarii*	rr. ventrales from nn. spinales	C1–L4
5.1.1	mm intertransversarii mediales lumborum	rr. ventrales from nn. spinales	Lateral bending of spine
5.1.2	mm. intertransversarii laterales lumborum	rr. ventrales from nn. spinales	Lateral bending of spine
5.1.3	mm. intertransversarii thoracis	rr. ventrales from nn. spinales	Lateral bending of spine

Table 5.6 (continued)

Muscle	Motor nerve	Motor neuron pool	Action
5.1.4　mm. intertransversarii anteriores cervicis	rr. ventrales from nn. spinales		Lateral bending of spine
5.1.5　mm intertransversarii posteriores cervicis 　　　pars medialis 　　　pars lateralis	rr. ventrales from nn. spinales		Lateral bending of spine
5.2　　*mm. interspinales*	rr. dorsales from nn. spinales	C1-L4	
5.2.1　mm. interspinales lumborum	rr. dorsales from nn. spinales		Extension of spine
5.2.2　mm. interspinales thoracis	rr. dorsales from nn. spinales		Extension of spine
5.2.3　mm. interspinales cervicis	rr. dorsales from nn. spinales		Extension of spine

muscles were called the posterolateral muscle group, including m. semi-spinalis capitis, m. longissimus capitis, m. splenius cervicis, m. levator scapulae, m. splenius capitis and m. trapezius. This subdivision has not been maintained. Laterally and posteriorly we now distinguish six main muscles: m. sternocleidomastoideus, m. transversospinalis, m. erector spi-nae, m. levator scapulae, m. splenius capitis and m. trapezius (Fig. 5.4).

It must be stressed that because of the large number of smaller muscles, the variability of CT scan pictures at the neck level tends to be more impor-tant than at other levels. A small deviation from the normal X-ray inci-dence can cause considerable variation in CT pictures.

5.2.2 The Shoulder Muscle Level

Our second CT scan makes a horizontal section through the shoulder muscles. The standard picture is taken with the patient in the supine posi-tion, with shoulders relaxed and arms at the sides. The focusing points used with different scanners are described in Table 5.1 and in Figs. 5.1 and 5.2. Posteriorly the CT scan cuts through the fossa infraspinata of the scapula and the vertebra T2 or T3. The radiological landmark of this level is the elongated linear appearance of the scapular shadow. At this level there is a sizeable distance between the scapula and the rib cage. This space is filled by the m. subscapularis, which at this level is approximately equal in size to the m. infraspinatus.

As can be seen in Figs. 5.5 and 5.6, the number of muscles visible is more restricted at this level than in the neck. They are, however, clinically more important because many neuromuscular diseases start as either a facio-scapulohumeral or a limb-girdle syndrome. The muscles at this level be-long to two major functional groups, those linking the shoulder to the trunk and those linking the shoulder to the upper extremity (Table 5.7). Some of the higher insertions of upper arm muscles (Table 5.8) can at times also be seen. Although we have not carried out this procedure ourselves, we want to mention that it is possible to improve on the definition of the different muscles at this level by creating a "subtrapezial space", by raising the arms of the patient above the head (THOMPSON and KREEL 1979). This procedure may be particularly interesting in the study of facioscapulohumeral syn-dromes.

5.2.3 The Abdominal Wall and Spinal Muscle Level

The third CT scan makes a horizontal section through the abdomen at ap-proximately the L4 level. The scan is again obtained with the patient in the

Table 5.7. Shoulder muscles

	Muscle	Motor nerve	Motor neu-ron pool	Action
1	*Shoulder-trunk muscles*			
1.1	*Posterior group*			
1.1.1	m. trapezius	n. accessorius (XI) and Branches of plexus cervicalis	nu. ambiguus C2-C4	Draws scapula towards spine Exorotation of scapula Draws shoulder upward Extension of head and bending of neck
1.1.2	m. latissimus dorsi	n. thoracodorsalis	C6-C8	Adduction and internal rotation of arm Drawing down raised arm Drawing down scapula Drawing back scapula
1.1.3	m. rhomboideus major	n. dorsalis scapulae	C4-C5	Draws scapula upward and medially Endorotates scapula Depresses shoulder
1.1.4	m. rhomboideus minor	n. dorsalis scapulae	C4-C5	Depresses shoulder
1.1.5	m. levator scapulae	n. dorsalis scapulae and branches of plexus cervicalis	C3-C5	Drawing scapula upward Bending neck laterally
1.2	*Anterior group*			
1.2.1	m. pectoralis major	Branches of plexus brachialis	C5-T1	Flexion and adduction of arm Internal rotation of arm Raising of ribs in forced inspiration

1.2.2	m. pectoralis minor	Branches of plexus brachialis	C7-C8	Pulling forward of scapula Pulling downward lateral angle of scapula Assistance in raising ribs
1.2.3	m. subclavius	n. subclavius	C5	Depresses clavicula Keeps clavicula against sternum Assists in forced inspiration
1.2.4	m. serratus anterior	n. thoracicus longus	C5-C7	drawing forward and laterally of scapula Assists in inspiration
2	*Shoulder-upper extremity muscles*			
2.1	m. deltoideus	n. axillaris	C5-C6	Abduction, flexion and extension of arm Internal and external rotation of arm
2.2	m. supraspinatus	n. suprascapularis	C5-C6	Abduction of arm Fixation of head of humerus during abduction
2.3	m. infraspinatus	n. suprascapularis	C5-C6	External rotation of arm against resistance (elbow being flexed)
2.4	m. teres minor	n. axillaris	C5-C6	Lateral rotation and adduction of arm
2.5	m. teres major	n. thoracodorsalis	C6-C7	Adduction, extension and medial rotation of arm
2.6	m. subscapularis	n. subscapularis	C5-C6	Internal rotation of humerus Adduction of humerus Fixation of head of humerus

Table 5.8. Upper-arm muscles

	Muscle	Motor nerve	Motor neuron pool	Action
1	*Flexor muscles*			
1.1	m. biceps brachii			
	caput longum	n. musculocutaneous	C5-C6	Flexion of elbow and shoulder
		n. musculocutaneous	C5-C6	Supination of forearm
				Fixation of forearm
	caput breve	n. musculocutaneous	C5-C6	Flexion of elbow and adduction at shoulder joint
1.2	m. coracobrachialis	n. musculocutaneous	C6-C7	Adduction and flexion in shoulder
1.3	m. brachialis	n. musculocutaneous	C5-C6	Flexion of forearm
				Flexion of arm against resistance
2	*Extensor muscles*			
2.1	m. triceps brachii	n. radialis	C6-C8	Extension of elbow joint
	caput longum			Adduction of arm
	caput mediale			Maintaining elbow in extended position
	caput laterale			

Table 5.9 Abdominal muscles (musculi abdominis)

	Muscle	Motor nerve	Motor neuron pool	Action
1	*Ventral abdominal muscles*			
1.1	*Straight abdominal muscles*			
1.1.1	m. rectus abdominis	nn. intercostales T1-T12	T7-T12	Flexion of spine Depression of thorax
1.1.2	m. pyramidalis	n. subcostalis	T12	Tenses linea alba
1.2	*Large abdominal muscles*			
1.2.1	m. obliquus externus abdominis	nn. intercostales T5-T12 n. iliohypogastricus	T5-T12 (L1)	Support of abdominal viscera Flexion of spine Rotation of spine towards opposite side
1.2.2	m. obliquus internus abdominis	nn. intercostales T8-T12 n. iliohypogastricus n. ilioinguinalis	T8-T12	Support of abdominal viscera Flexion and abduction of spine Depression of thorax Flexion and rotation of pelvis
1.2.3	m. transversus abdominis	nn. intercostales T1-L1 n. iliohypogastricus n. ilioinguinalis	T7-L1	Support of abdominal viscera
2	*Dorsal abdominal muscles*			
2.1	m. quadratus lumborum	n. subcostalis Plexus lumbalis	T12-L3	Abduction and extension of spine Depression of rib 12

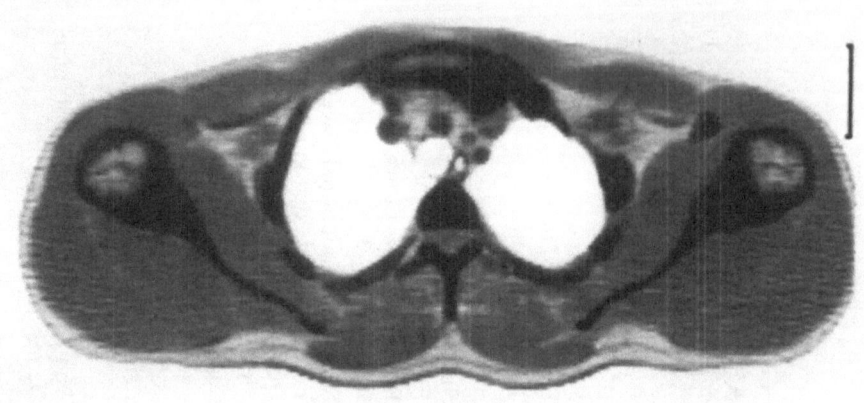

Fig. 5.5. Standard CT scan of the normal shoulder musculature. Bar = 5 cm

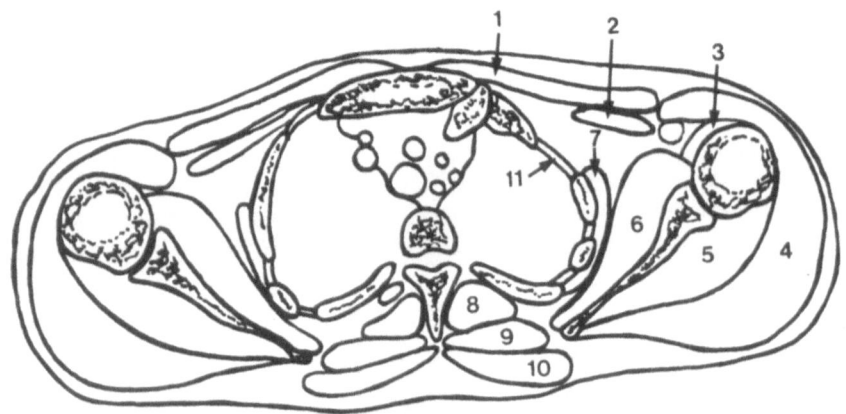

Fig. 5.6. Line drawing of the CT scan shown in Fig. 5.5. *1*, m. pectoralis major; *2*, m. pectoralis minor; *3*, m. biceps brachii, caput breve; *4*, m. deltoideus; *5*, m. infraspinatus; *6*, m. subscapularis; *7*, m. serratus anterior; *8*, m. transversospinalis, m. erector spinae; *9*, m. rhomboideus major; *10*, m. trapezius; *11*, mm. intercostales

supine position. The focusing point is slightly (1 cm) above a line connecting the upper edges of the cristae iliacae which corresponds to spinal level L4. In some subjects it may correspond to the level of the umbilicus. The radiological characteristic of this level is the large size of m. psoas major. The parameters of this scan are summarized in Table 5.1 and in Figs. 5.1 and 5.2.

As can be observed in Figs. 5.7 and 5.8, this section also contains muscles from different functional and anatomical groups. First some of the abdominal muscles (Table 5.9) can be seen. On the other hand, the m.

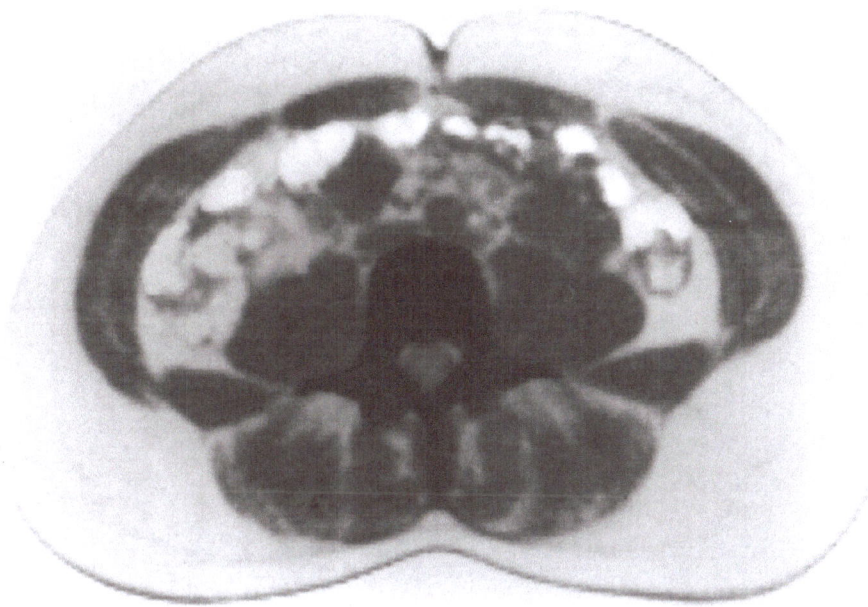

Fig. 5.7. Standard CT scan of the normal abdominal and spinal muscles

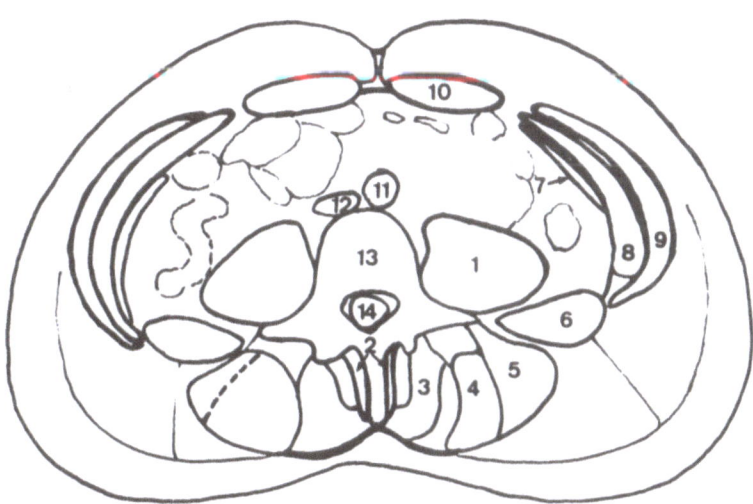

Fig. 5.8. Line drawing of CT scan shown in Fig. 5.7. *1*, m. psoas major; *2* (*arrows*), m. interspinalis; *3*, m. multifidus; *4*, m. longissimus; *5*, m. iliocostalis; *6*, m. quadratus lumborum; *7* (*arrow*), m. transversus abdominis; *8*, m. obliquus internus abdominis; *9*, m. obliquus externus abdominis; *10*, m. rectus abdominis; *11*, aorta abdominalis; *12*, vena cava inferior; *13*, vertebra L4; *14*, medulla spinalis

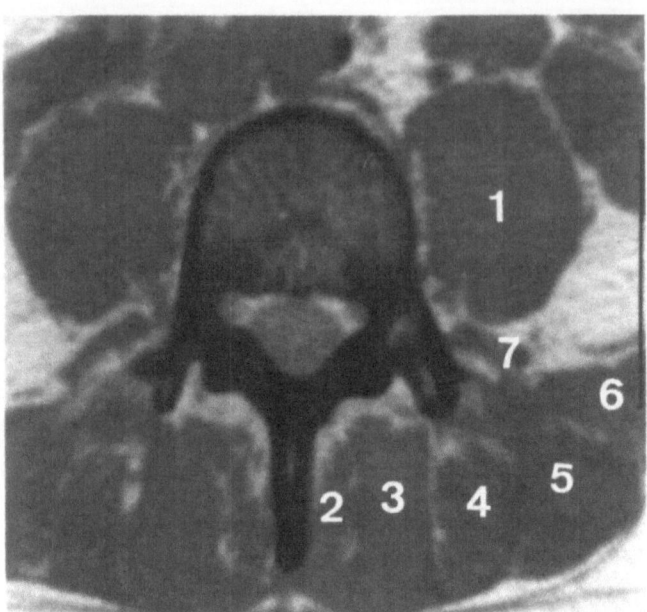

Fig. 5.9. Enlargement of mm. dorsi at level L4. *1*, m. psoas major; *2*, m. interspinalis; *3*, m. multifidus; *4*, m. longissimus; *5*, m. intercostalis; *6*, m. quadratus lumborum; *7*, m. intertransversarius lateralis et medialis. Bar = 5 cm

psoas major, which is the largest single muscle at this level, belongs anatomically to the pelvic muscles described in Table 5.10. Posteriorly, the lumbar component of the extensor muscles of the spine (mm. dorsi; summarized in Table 5.6) can be seen.

Although the clinical examination of muscles at this level is usually neglected, they form a group of very great functional significance. In some figures it is amazing to see how small the abdominal cavity really is, compared with large blocks of muscle. The abdominal wall muscles support the viscera, and atrophy and paralysis of those muscles is largely responsible for the pseudo-obesity observed in many patients with neuromuscular diseases. The m. psoas major and the mm. dorsi, on the other hand, are of utmost importance for maintaining the erect position of the spine and its normal curvature. They form a highly balanced system of agonists and antagonists which is disturbed sooner or later in a large number of neuromuscular diseases (Fig. 5.9). It is very unfortunate that this level has only recently been added to the standard examination procedure.

5.2.4 The Pelvic Muscle Level

The fourth CT scan of the standard examination procedure makes a horizontal section through the pelvic muscles. Although these form a rather homogeneous anatomical and functional group (Table 5.10), the higher insertions of several muscles which anatomically belong to the thigh muscles (Table 5.11) can also be observed. Variation at this level is rather limited except for the differences in male and female anatomy.

A standard CT scan of the pelvic muscles is demonstrated in Figs. 5.10 and 5.11. The scan is carried out with the patient in the supine position. The focusing point is the middle of the symphysis pubica. The radiological characteristics are the three well-separated shadows of the symphysis pubica anteriorly, the os femoris laterally and the os ischii posteriorly. The radiographic parameters are summarized in Table 5.1. With earlier scanners, however, we focused on the middle of the ligamentum inguinale, producing a different picture which shows more of the mm. glutei. This has been represented separately in Figs. 5.12 and 5.13, because many clinical scans have been taken at this level.

The pelvic muscles are clinically of utmost importance. Very many neuromuscular diseases start as lower limb-girdle syndromes. Furthermore, many muscles at this level cannot be approached by any other technical means such as analytical muscular power testing or EMG. This is particularly the case for such important muscles as the m. iliopsoas and mm. obturatorii internus and externus which play an important role in maintaining upright position and normal gait.

5.2.5 The Thigh Muscle Level

The fifth CT scan of the standard examination procedure makes a horizontal section through the thigh muscles summarized in Table 5.11. Almost all muscles of this group can be visualized on the standard CT scan.

A standard CT scan of the thigh muscles is demonstrated in Figs. 5.14 and 5.15. The focusing point is a line 15 cm above the upper edge of the patella (Fig. 5.1).

The clinical importance of this group must be stressed. Clinically it is of utmost importance in maintaining normal gait. Above all, however, we found the thigh muscles to offer an excellent model for examining the relationship between radiological parameters such as muscle density and size and muscle strength as tested by analytical muscular testing. In addition, very specific patterns of atrophy and/or hypertrophy have been observed at this level, allowing for a detailed study of the relationship between the processes of atrophy and hypertrophy and the underlying patho-anatomical parameters.

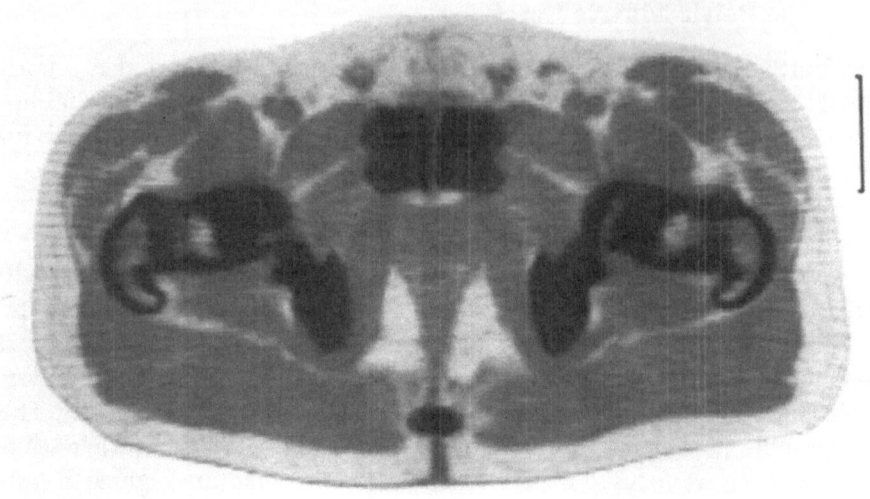

Fig. 5.10. Standard CT scan of the normal pelvic muscles. Bar = 5 cm

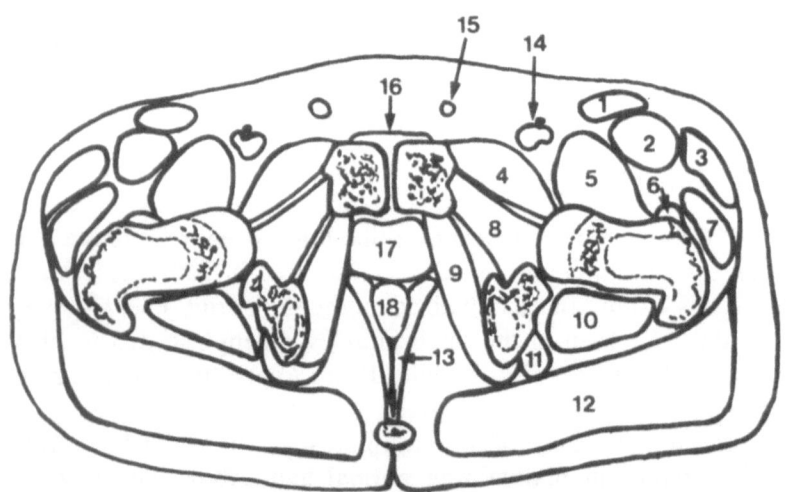

Fig. 5.11. Line drawing of the CT scan shown in Fig. 5.10. *1*, m. sartorius; *2*, m. rectus femoris; *3*, m. tensor fasciae latae; *4*, m. adductor magnus, m. pectineus; *5*, m. iliopsoas; *6*, m. vastus lateralis; *7*, m. gluteus medius; *8*, m. obturatorius externus; *9*, m. obturatorius internus; *10*, m. quadratus femoris; *11*, m. semimembranosus; *12*, m. gluteus maximus; *13*, m. levator ani; *14*, nervus, arteria, vena femoralis; *15*, ductus spermaticus; *16*, ligamentum suspensorium penis; *17*, vesica urinaria, prostata; *18*, rectum

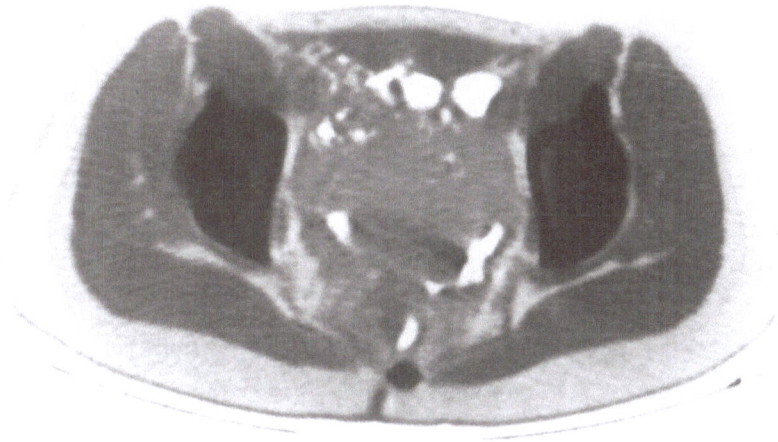

Fig. 5.12. CT scan of the normal pelvic muscles through the middle of ligamentum inguinale (focus 4.1 in Fig. 5.1)

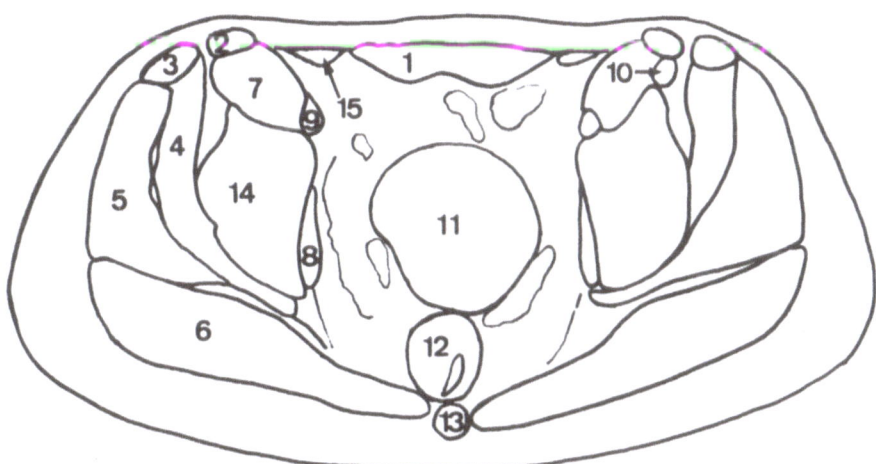

Fig. 5.13. Line drawing of CT scan shown in Fig. 5.12. *1,* mm. recti abdominis; *2,* m. sartorius; *3,* m. tensor fasciae latae; *4,* m. gluteus minimus; *5,* m. gluteus medius; *6,* m. gluteus maximus; *7,* m. iliopsoas; *8,* m. obturatorius internus; *9,* neurovascular bundle; *10,* m. rectus femoris; *11,* vesica urinaria; *12,* rectum; *13,* os sacrum; *14,* articulatio coxae; *15,* ligamentum inguinale, canalis inguinalis

Table 5.10. Pelvic muscles

	Muscle	Motor nerve	Motor neu-ron pool	Action
1	*Internal pelvic muscles*			
1.1	m. iliopsoas			
1.1.1	m. psoas major	Branches of plexus lumbalis n. femoralis	L1-L4	Tilting of thigh at hip joint Rotation of thigh Flexion of spine and pelvis Abduction of lumbar part of spine
1.1.2	m. iliacus	Branches of plexus lumbalis n. femoralis	L1-L4	Flexion and external rotation of thigh at hip joint with flexed leg Forward tilting of pelvis
2	*External pelvic muscles*			
2.1	m. gluteus maximus	n. gluteus inferior	L5-S2	Extension and external rotation of thigh Tension of fascia lata and iliotibial band Keeps extended knee joint steady
2.2	m. gluteus medius	n. gluteus superior	L4-S1	Abduction and extension of thigh External rotation (posterior part) Internal rotation (anterior part)
2.3	m. piriformis	Branches of plexus sacralis	S1-S2	Abduction and external rotation of thigh Extension of thigh
2.4	m. obturatorius internus	Plexus sacralis	L5-S2	External rotation of thigh Extension and abduction of flexed thigh

2.5	mm. gemelli			
2.5.1	m. gemellus superior	Plexus sacralis	L4-S1	External rotation of thigh Extension and abduction of flexed thigh
2.5.2	m. gemellus inferior	Plexus sacralis	L4-S1	External rotation of thigh Extension and abduction of flexed thigh
2.6	m. quadratus femoris	Plexus sacralis	L4-S1	External rotation and abduction of thigh
2.7	m. obturatorius externus	n. obturatorius	L3-L4	External rotation and adduction of thigh Fixation of head of femur
2.8	m. gluteus minimus	n. gluteus superior	L4-S1	Abduction of thigh Internal rotation (anterior part) of thigh Flexion (anterior part) and extension (posterior part) of thigh

Table 5.11. Thigh muscles

	Muscle	Motor nerve	Motor neuron pool	Action
1	*Anterior thigh muscles*			
1.1	m. sartorius	n. femoralis	L2-L3	Flexion of thigh at hip joint
				Abduction and external rotation of thigh
				Flexion and internal rotation of leg
				Tenses fascia lata
1.2	m. quadriceps femoris	n. femoralis	L2-L4	
1.2.1	m. rectus femoris			Flexion of thigh at hip joint
				Extension of leg
1.2.2	m. vastus lateralis			Extension of knee
1.2.3	m. vastus medialis			Extension of knee
1.2.4	m. vastus intermedius			Extension of knee
2	*Medial thigh muscles*			
2.1	m. pectineus	n. femoralis	L2-L3	Adduction and flexion of thigh
		n. obturatorius		External rotation (foot off ground)
2.2	m. gracilis	n. obturatorius	L2-L4	Adduction and flexion of thigh
				External rotation of thigh
2.3	m. adductor longus	n. obturatorius	L2-L3	Adduction and flexion of thigh (external rotation)
2.4	m. adductor brevis	n. obturatorius	L2-L4	Adduction and flexion of thigh (external rotation)

2.5	m. adductor magnus	n. obturatorius (linea aspera part) n. tibialis (epicondylus medialis part)	L3-L4	Adduction of thigh, flexion and external rotation of thigh (superior and middle part) Extension (inferior part) of thigh
3	*Dorsal thigh muscles*			
3.1	m. semitendinosus	n. tibialis	L4-S1	Extension and adduction of thigh Internal rotation of thigh Flexion of leg Internal rotation of leg (knee flexed)
3.2	m. semimembranosus	n. tibialis	L4-S1	Internal rotation and flexion of leg Extension and adduction of thigh Internal rotation of thigh
3.3	m. biceps femoris			
3.3.1	caput longum	n. tibialis	L5-S1	Extension and adduction of thigh Flexion of leg External rotation of leg
3.3.2	caput breve	n. peroneus communis	L5-S1	Extension and adduction of thigh Flexion of leg
4	*Lateral thigh muscles*			
4.1	m. tensor fasciae latae	n. gluteus superior	L4-L5	Flexion, internal rotation and abduction of thigh Flexion, abduction and external rotation of pelvis External rotation of tibia

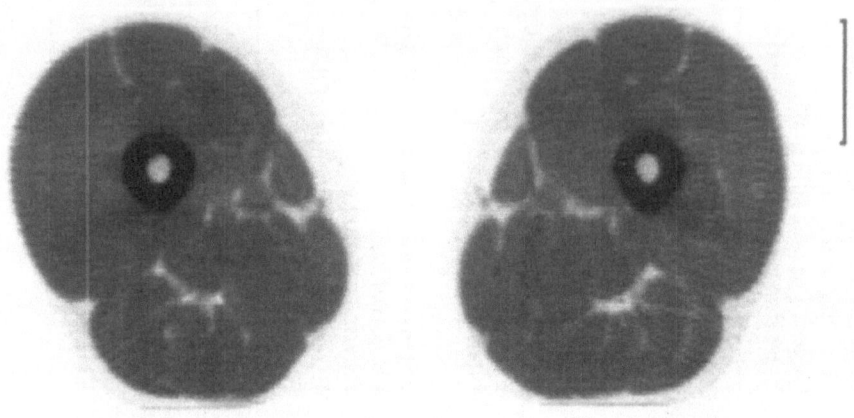

Fig. 5.14. Standard CT scan of the normal thigh muscles. Bar = 5 cm

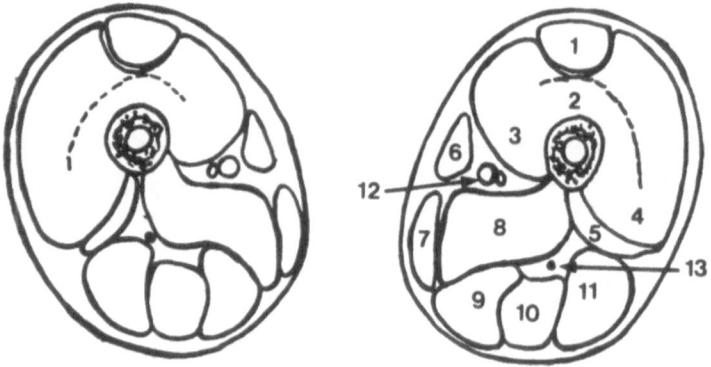

Fig. 5.15. Line drawing of the CT scan shown in Fig. 5.14. *1*, m. rectus femoris; *2*, m. vastus intermedius; *3*, m. vastus medialis; *4*, m. vastus lateralis; *5*, m. biceps femoris, caput breve; *6*, m. sartorius; *7*, m. gracilis; *8*, m. adductor magnus; *9*, m. semimembranosus; *10*, m. semitendinosus; *11*, m. biceps femoris, caput longum; *12*, a. and v. femoralis; *13*, n. ischiadicus; *9, 10* and *11* together form the so-called hamstrings

5.2.6 The Lower Leg Muscle Level

The sixth and final CT scan (Fig. 5.16) makes a horizontal section through the lower leg muscles. Here again the CT scan visualizes all muscles of the functional and anatomical group of lower leg muscles described in Table 5.12. But, especially at this level it can be seen that normality and good anatomy are inversely proportional to each other. A line drawing here is

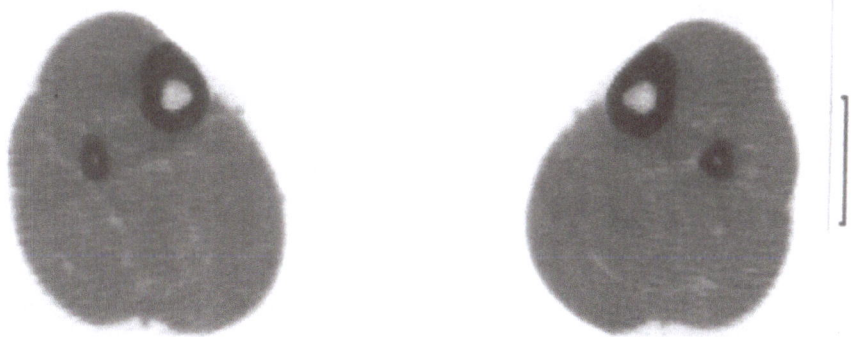

Fig. 5.16. Standard CT scan of the normal lower leg muscles. Bar = 5 cm

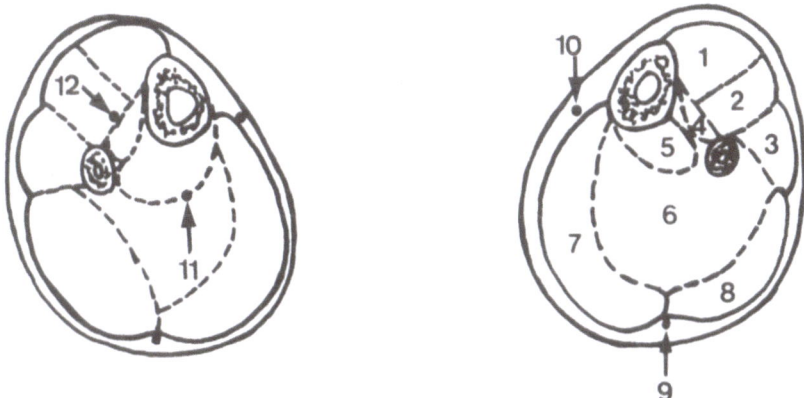

Fig. 5.17. Line drawing of the CT scan shown in Fig. 5.16. *1*, m. tibialis anterior; *2*, m. extensor digitorum longus, m. hallucis longus; *3*, m. peroneus longus, m. peroneus brevis; *4*, m. tibialis posterior; *5*, m. popliteus, m. flexor digitorum longus; *6*, m. soleus; *7*, m. gastrocnemius, caput mediale; *8*, m. gastrocnemius, caput laterale; *9*, vena saphena parva; *10*, vena saphena magna; *11*, n. tibialis; *12*, n. peroneus profundus

mandatory (Fig. 5.17) to retrieve the muscles as they are seen in pathological scans. When the muscles are normal, almost no anatomical details can be seen.

Visualization of the lower leg muscles is of particular interest because they are the only group of distal muscles in the standard examination procedure. As explained previously, the distal muscles of the upper extremities cannot be adequately examined. Not many neuromuscular diseases start with distal muscle involvement, as does dystrophia myotonica, but all eventually do affect these muscles. Each initial distal muscle involvement can therefore be of diagnostic significance. Furthermore, some of the most

Table 5.12 Lower leg muscles

Muscle	Motor nerve	Motor neuron pool	Action
1 Anterior muscle group			
1.1 m. tibialis anterior	n. peroneus profundus	L4-S1	Dorsiflexion of foot at ankle joint Inversion of foot (foot dorsiflexed)
1.2 m. extensor hallucis longus	n. peroneus profundus	L4-S1	Dorsiflexion of foot at ankle joint Extension of great toe
1.3 m. extensor digitorum longus	n. peroneus profundus	L4-S1	Dorsiflexion of foot at ankle joint Extension at metacarpophalangeal and interphalangeal joints II to V Slight eversion of foot
2 Lateral muscle group			
2.1 m. peroneus longus	n. peroneus superficialis	L5-S1	Dorsiflexion and abduction of foot Eversion of foot
2.2 m. peroneus brevis	n. peroneus superficialis	L5-S1	Eversion of foot (plantar flexion of foot)
3 Dorsal muscle group			
3.1 Superficial layer			
3.1 m. triceps surae			
3.1.1 m. gastrocnemius			Plantar flexion and supination of foot Flexion of knee Raising of heel

3.1.1.1	caput mediale	n. tibialis	L5-S2	Plantar flexion of foot at ankle joint Raising of heel
3.1.1.2	caput laterale	n. tibialis	L5-S2	Raising of heel
3.1.2	m. soleus	n. tibialis	L5-S2	Plantar flexion of foot at ankle joint Raising of heel
3.1.3	m. plantaris	n. tibialis	L4-S1	Flexion of leg at knee joint
3.2	*Deep layer*			
3.2.1	m. popliteus	n. tibialis	L4-S1	Internal rotation of leg
3.2.2	m. flexor digitorum longus	n. tibialis	L5-S2	Flexion of phalanges of four lateral toes Supination and flexion of foot at ankle joint Support of longitudinal foot arches
3.2.3	m. tibialis posterior	n. tibialis	L5-S1	Inversion of foot Support of foot arches (plantar flexion of foot)
3.2.4	m. flexor hallucis longus	n. tibialis	L5-S2	Flexion of phalanges of great toe Plantar flexion and supination of foot Support of longitudinal foot arches

remarkable features of neuromuscular diseases such as the pseudo-hypertrophy of Duchenne and Becker dystrophies are seen in these muscles. Finally, as described in the previous level, very peculiar patterns of atrophy and hypertrophy are observed here which allow for interesting correlative studies between radiological and pathological parameters.

5.3 Marker Muscles

As we have described, it has been necessary to limit the examination of the skeletal muscular system to a number of well-selected target areas in order to make it clinically useful. Because we also sought to take advantage of the possibilities which CT scanners provide to obtain numerical values for certain parameters of the skeletal muscular system such as muscle size and density, a selection was made of a small number of muscles or muscle

Table 5.13. Marker muscles

Level			Marker muscles
1	Neck muscles	1.1	m. sternocleidomastoideus
		1.2	m. transversospinalis
2	Shoulder muscles	2.1	m. deltoideus
		2.2	m. subscapularis
		2.3	m. infraspinatus
3	Abdominal wall and spinal muscles	3.1	m. psoas major
		3.2	mm. dorsi
4	Pelvic muscles	4.1	m. gluteus maximus
		4.2	m. iliopsoas
5	Thigh muscles	5.1	*m. quadriceps*
			m. rectus femoris
			m. vastus lateralis
			m. vastus intermedius
			m. vastus medialis
		5.2	m. sartorius
		5.3	m. gracilis
		5.4	m. biceps femoris (caput breve)
6	Lower leg muscles	6.1	*m. triceps surae*
			m. soleus
			m. gastrocnemius
			(caput mediale)
			(caput laterale)
			m. tibialis anterior

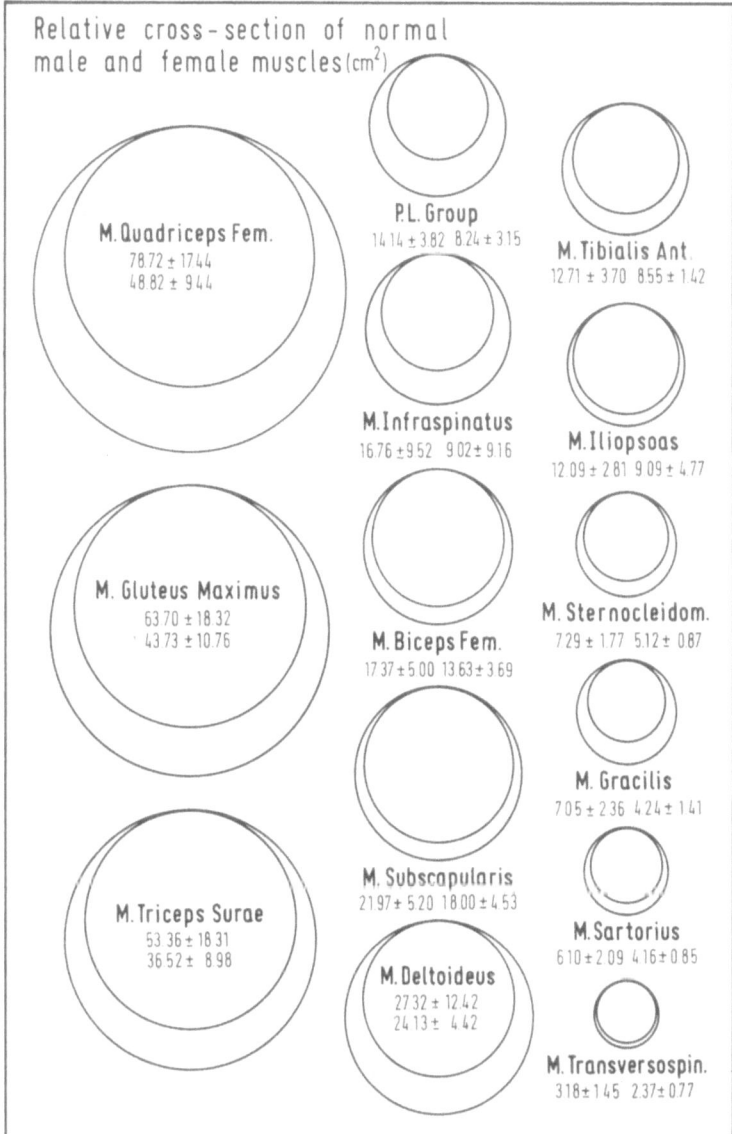

Fig. 5.18. Relative cross section of normal male and female muscles. The surface area of a number of muscles (marker muscles) was measured on 15 normal males and 15 normal females. The mean surface area was then calculated and represented as a circular surface. The *outer circle* of each represents the male muscle, the *inner circle* the female muscle. The *upper figures* within the circles represent the mean value of the surface area ± 1 SD for males, the *lower figures* represent the mean ± 1 SD for females

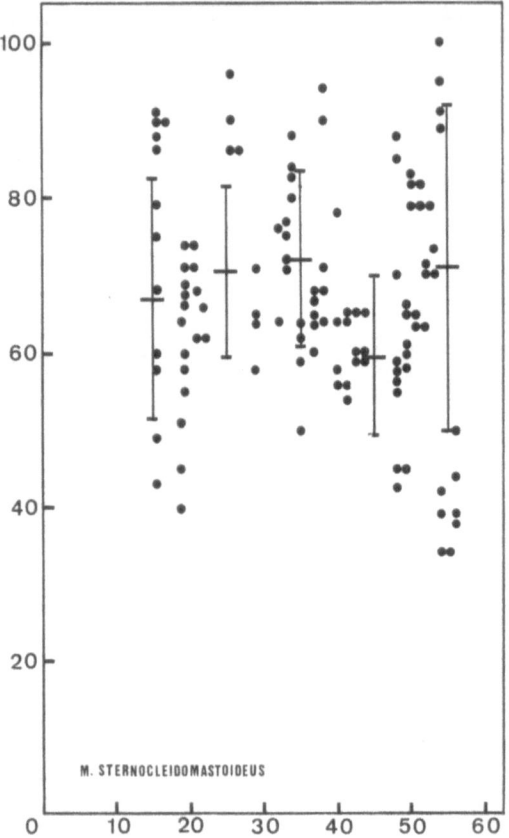

Fig. 5.19. Density measurements on m. sternocleidomastoideus of normal persons of different age groups, measured with different scanners. The bar graphs represent the mean value ± 1 SD for the pooled data of each age group

groups which we called "marker muscles". Numerical data acquisition was limited to these muscles, which are summarized in Table 5.13.

The selection criteria for marker muscles were their consistent and distinctive presence in all pictures obtained of a certain scan level, and a sufficiently large size that reliable measurements of surface and density parameters were possible. Marker muscles were also selected so that together they represented a large sample of motor neuron pools on a significant number of spinal cord levels. Some were selected because biopsies are frequently taken of them, or because they have been well studied, particularly in relation to their fibre-type composition (see Table 2.1). Finally, most marker muscles were found to be interesting for study in pathological scans because of either selective or peculiar muscular atrophy of hypertrophy.

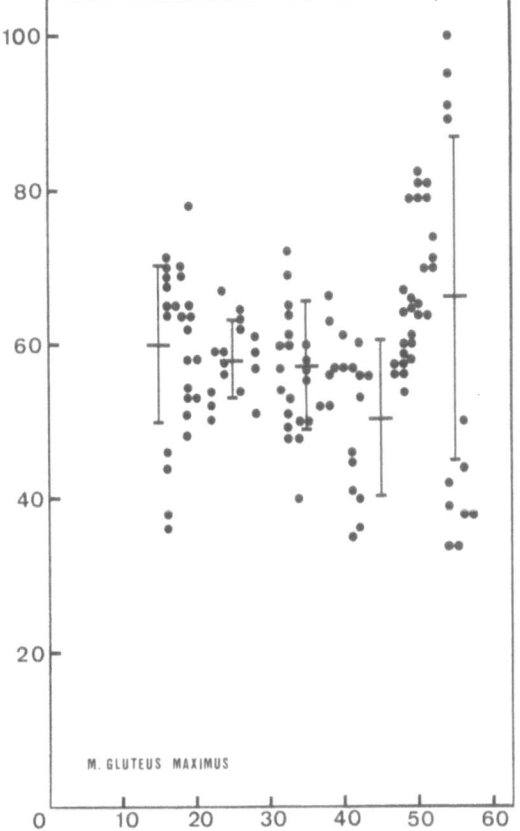

Fig. 5.20. Density measurements on m. gluteus maximus represented as described for Fig. 5.19

For each of the marker muscles numerical values of normal size and density have been determined on a group of males and females of different ages without symptoms or signs of muscular disease. Values of relative cross sections of a group of muscles measured in 30 patients are presented in Fig. 5.18. It is obvious that the muscles which are responsible for erect posture and gait are by far the largest of the body, and that there is a consistent difference between male and female muscles. Unfortunately, we were not able to extend these data because scan levels were changed and because one of the scanners did not have the necessary program built in. Data on normal density measurements of human skeletal muscles are presented in Figs. 5.19 and 5.20. Here, the program initially started on a slow scanner, could be supplemented by new data on a fast scanner.

6 Basic Radiological Changes in Diseased Skeletal Muscle

In this chapter, four basic radiological changes which can be observed by CT scanning in diseased skeletal muscle will be described. They are (1) muscular atrophy, (2) muscular hypertrophy, (3) muscular hypotrophy and (4) muscular fibrosis. It will be shown that these basic morphological changes can be observed either alone or in combination with each other at various stages of different disease processes without being specific for any of them. For example, muscular atrophy can be seen in combination with hypertrophy of synergistic muscles. It can produce pseudohypertrophy or lead to muscular hypotrophy. Fibrosis can be observed as a separate entity but can also occur together with muscular atrophy.

Many examples in this chapter were selected from pelvic muscles and the lower extremities, because they could best be observed in this area and because of the homogeneity of the presentation. The same basic lesions, however, were also found on the other levels which were examined.

6.1 Muscular Atrophy

In most neuromuscular diseases, whether the lesion be in the lower motor neuron, the peripheral axon, the neuromuscular junction or the muscle itself, the muscle cells will sooner or later undergo irreversible atrophy. When the regenerative capacity of the muscle (MAURO 1979) can no longer keep pace with this atrophy, the total number of muscle cells will decrease. In most cases, the area of the degenerated muscle fibres will then be invaded by other tissue elements. Pathological studies (ADAMS 1975) have demonstrated that ultimately tissue will be replaced mainly by fat cells, together with a variable amount of reticular fibrils and collagen in perimysia and aponeuroses. Therefore, the radiological expression of muscular atrophy in all diseases studied so far by CT scanning consists in the appearance of low-density areas in the skeletal muscles. Depending on the amount of tissue replacement, the size of the muscular mass may remain the same, decrease or increase.

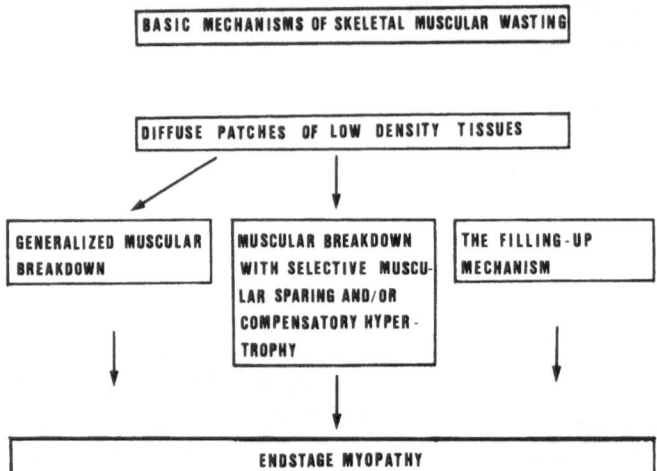

Fig. 6.1. Scheme of the three main pathways of skeletal muscular breakdown

Two main features of muscular atrophy will be described. First, from the presently available morphological information obtained by CT scanning, muscular atrophy can be reconstructed as a number of continuous processes along several different lines of progression. Secondly, attention will be focused on one of the most striking findings about muscular atrophy – its remarkable selectivity – which can be found between groups of muscles, between individual muscles and even between parts of compound muscles such as the m. quadriceps.

Although we have not yet conducted a follow-up in any one patient long enough to fully confirm our findings, muscular atrophy seems to progress along three main lines (Fig. 6.1). The first two are characterized by an initial stage in which small patches of low-density tissue appear within the muscles. In some diseases, e.g. myasthenia gravis, the process may remain at this stage for a long time or the muscle may even return to normal. In others, however, the process may continue in one of two ways. Either the muscles will progressively break down into more and more ragged configurations, with small remnants of muscle finally dispersed within large areas of fat tissue, or the atrophy can proceed in concurrence with very pronounced compensatory hypertrophy of synergistic muscles. The first process seems to occur predominantly in spinal muscular atrophies while the second is seen most frequently in muscular dystrophies. A third type of atrophy seems to start with small areas of fat infiltration, usually well circumscribed at the edge of the muscles, inside the fascia, followed by a progressive filling-up of this fascia with fat. This third type also seems to occur most frequently in muscular dystrophies. All types of atrophy may finally lead to an end-stage in which practically all muscles have disappeared.

6.1.1 Muscular Atrophy as a Continuous Process

6.1.1.1 Small Patches of Low-Density Tissue

The first sign of muscular atrophy is usually the appearance, diffusely dispersed within one or several muscles, of small dots of low-density tissue, giving the muscles a "vacuolar" or "moth-eaten" appearance. The original muscular mass remains normally circumscribed, without any significant contour damage and without any sizeable loss of mass within the original fascia (Fig. 6.2). At this stage it is not possible to make a differential diagnosis between muscular atrophy due to progressive myopathies such as muscular dystrophies, atrophy of spinal or peripheral neurogenic origin and disuse atrophy. Only the initial stages of two immunological diseases, polymyositis and myasthenia gravis, seem to differ. In these diseases the small patches of low-density tissue seem to be more linear and slightly mor extensive from the onset. They may correspond more to myo-oedema and inflammatory infiltrate than to muscular atrophy in the case of polymyositis (Fig. 6.3) and to lymphocyte infiltration in the case of myasthenia gravis (Fig. 6.4). A differential diagnosis between pure atrophy and atrophy mixed with myo-oedema or infiltrate has been attempted by employing intravenous contrast media in myasthenia gravis, as will be described further.

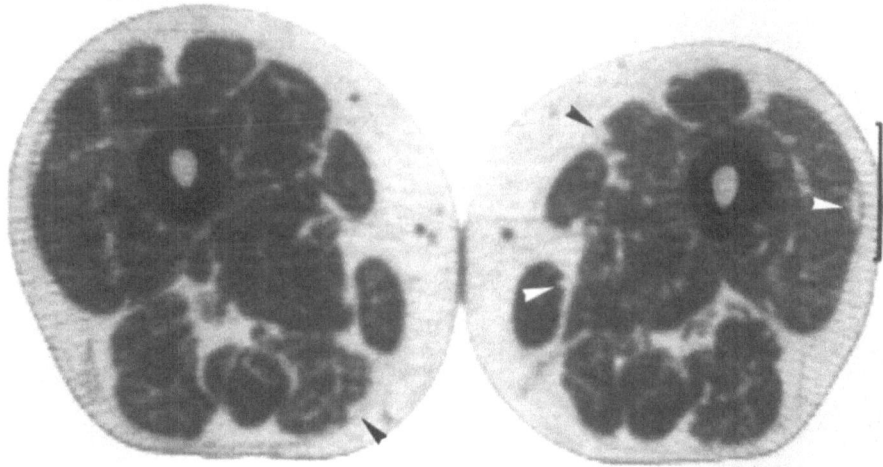

Fig. 6.2. First stage of skeletal muscular wasting in a 49-year-old male with disuse atrophy due to long-standing immobilization: diffuse and homogeneous infiltration of small patches of low-density tissue in all muscles. Some of these patches are situated immediately below the fascia, giving the impression of fascia breakdown (*arrows*). Bar = 5 cm

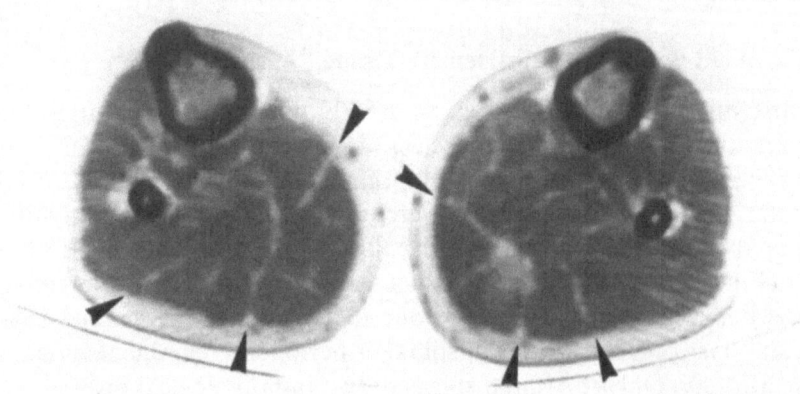

Fig. 6.3. Initial stage of atrophy in the lower legs of a 40-year-old patient with chronic polymyositis. The low-density tissue has a coarser linear aspect (*arrows*), possibly due to inflammatory infiltrate or to lymphocyte infiltration in the case of myasthenia gravis as shown in Fig. 6.4

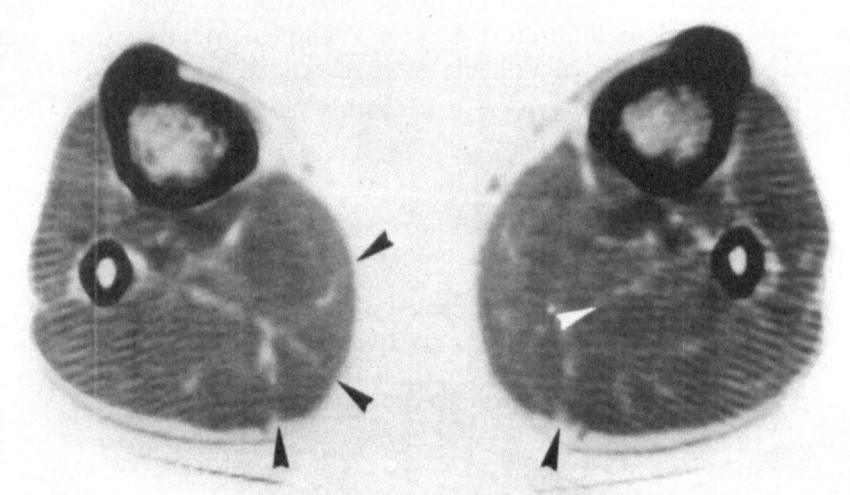

Fig. 6.4. Initial stage of atrophy in a 60-year-old patient with myasthenia gravis. Very similar findings to those in Fig. 6.3, probably diagnostic

6.1.1.2 The Muscular Breakdown Mechanism

Particularly in spinal muscular atrophies, but also in other diseases such as polymyositis and amyotrophic lateral sclerosis, this initial stage of small patches of low-density tissue is followed by a series of steps which eventually lead to total wasting of all muscles. The two main characteristics of this

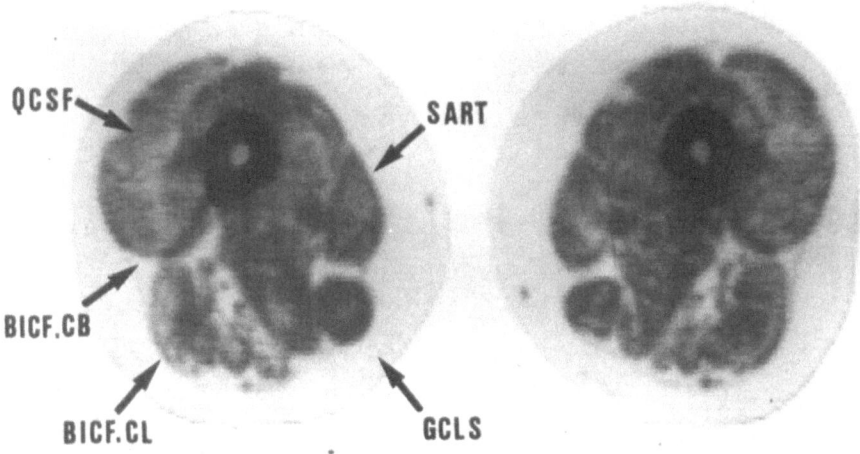

Fig. 6.5. Dominant distal muscular dystrophy in a 24-year-old female. Probably due to confluence of the small low-density tissue patches, the muscles acquire a "cloudy" appearance. Selectivity already becomes apparent at this stage. The deeper layer of m. quadriceps femoris (*QCSF*) is more affected than the superficial layer, the caput breve of m. biceps femoris (*BICF.CB*) is well preserved in contrast to the caput longum (*BICF.CL*), and m. sartoirus (*SART*) and m. gracilis (*GCLS*) are dense and hypertrophic

type of evolution are the progressively more ragged appearance of the muscles and the minimal compensatory hypertrophy compared with other diseases such as the X-linked muscular dystrophies.

It seems that one of the first things to happen is the increase and conflu ence of the small low-density tissue patches into larger fields, giving a progressively more "cloudy" appearance to the musculature (Fig. 6.5). The next step seems to be a breakdown of the muscular contours, producing an increasingly ragged configuration of the muscles, which finally retreat into small islands of tissue within a large panniculus adiposus (Fig. 6.6). It seems evident that in such cases fasciculations, if they are still present, will no longer be visible on the skin and that the conventional EMG needles are probably not long enough to reach into the muscular tissue itself; longer ones should be produced, if technically feasible, to examine such cases. These are also the cases in which it is, in fact, sometimes possible to "hear" the enlarged motor units by means of a standard stethoscope applied over the slightly contracting muscles (FREDERICKS and RUSSMAN 1979).

The ragged patterns and the small islands of muscle shown in Fig. 6.6 can be considered pathognomonic for spinal muscular atrophies (s.m.a.). In myopathies the muscular breakdown is usually more homogeneous (Fig. 6.7) than in s.m.a.

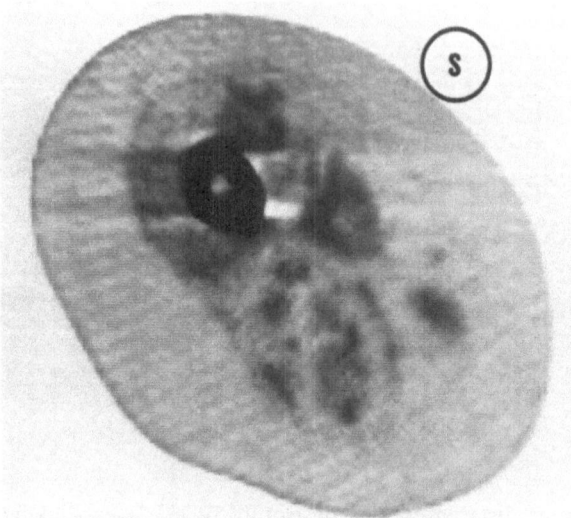

Fig. 6.6. Spinal muscular atrophy of the KUGELBERG-WELANDER (1956) type in a 28-year-old female. The muscles are totally broken up into small islands of ragged muscular tissue in a large panniculus adiposus. This can be considered pathognomonic for late stages of this disease. Attention is drawn to the possibility of hearing with a stethoscope (S) the rumbling noise of the enlarged motor units contracting within the "empty" thigh

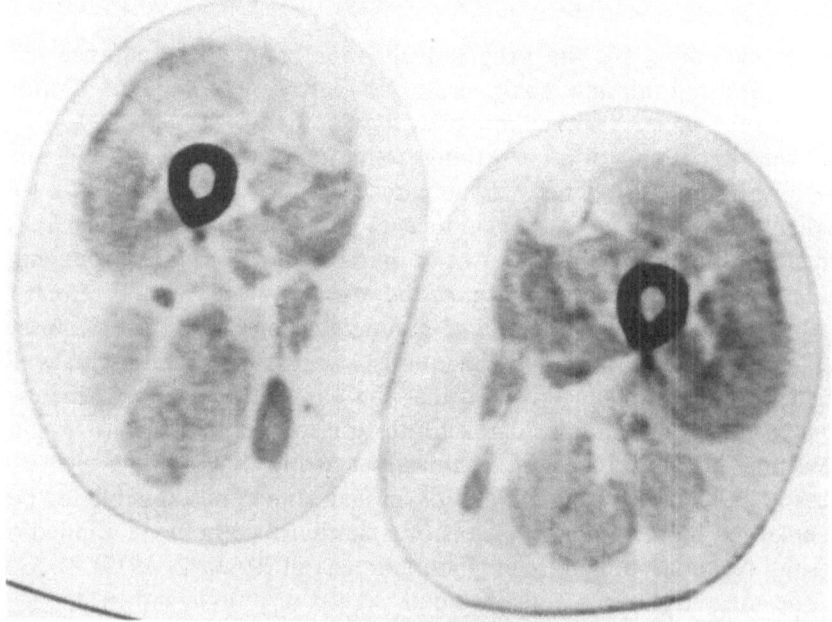

Fig. 6.7. Diffuse muscular breakdown without selectivity or compensatory mechanisms in a 10-year-old girl with a congenital myopathy of not yet determined aetiology

6.1.1.3 Muscular Breakdown with Compensatory Hypertrophy

A completely different picture can be observed in other myopathies. After the initial stage, selective atrophy occurs in one or more muscles or parts of muscles of a synergistic functional group. While the atrophy progresses, the remaining muscles or parts of muscles which carry the additional work load of the atrophic muscles are seen to undergo what is usually called compensatory hypertrophy, so that a mosaic pattern emerges, consisting of more or less strongly hypertrophic and more or less atrophic muscles. Some of the many examples of this phenomenon which have been observed in our series are represented in Figs. 6.8–6.12. Very frequently seen are compensatory hypertrophy of the m. rectus femoris in cases of m. quadriceps atrophy; the hypertrophy of one of the hamstring muscles, the m. semimembranosus, m. semitendinosus or m. biceps, in cases in which one of them underwent atrophy; and the hypertrophy of the m. sartorius and/or m. gracilis, mainly in cases of atrophy of the mm. adductores. Severel combinations have been observed, and in most cases the patterns are difficult to explain and unpredictable. Mixed patterns of atrophic and hypertrophic muscles can remain stable for a long time and allow the patient a remarkably good functional status. At later stages of the disease however, the spared muscles also undergo atrophy, functional handicaps appear and the patient gradually develops an end-stage myopathy (Fig. 6.12).

6.1.1.4 The "Filling-up" Process

In other diseases muscular atrophy seems to proceed in still another way. Within the intact muscular fascia, progressively more muscular tissue is replaced by low-density tissue, while the rest of the muscular mass remains fairly well preserved and the outline of the original muscular fascia remains clearly visible. This process, which can be observed mainly in muscular dystrophies, seems to start with small, well-circumscribed islands of fat, usually at the edge of the muscle mass just inside the fascia (Fig. 6.13). Larger areas of fat infiltration can then be formed, and finally the original muscle mass is totally filled with fat tissue (Figs. 6.14–6.16). It is clear that in such cases muscular atrophy does not coincide with clinically visible or measurable muscular hypotrophy. Here, muscular atrophy seems to consist merely in an exchange of active muscle cells by inactive connective tissue cells, altering the function but not the size of the original muscle. At no time during such an evolution is a significant degree of musclar wasting, as we have described previously, to be seen.

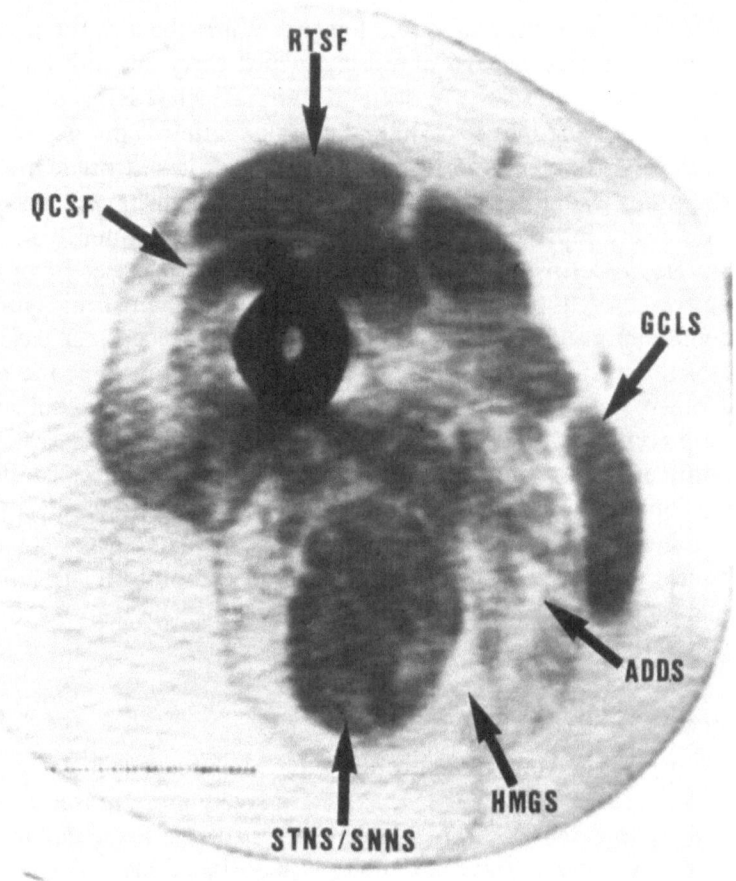

Fig. 6.8. Muscular atrophy with compensatory hypertrophy in a 48-year-old female with an autosomal recessive limb-girdle myopathy of not yet determined aetiology (limb-girdle dystrophy). Most muscles are severely wasted and in particular the m. quadriceps femoris (*QCSF*), the mm. adductores (*ADDS*) and the hamstring muscles (*HMGS*). Compensatory hypertrophy is seen in m. rectus femoris (*RTSF*), m. semitendinosus (*STNS*) and/or m. semimembranosus (*SNNS*). M. gracilis (*GCLS*) is well preserved but probably not hypertrophic. The thick panniculus adiposus prevents transcutaneous clinical appraisal of these events

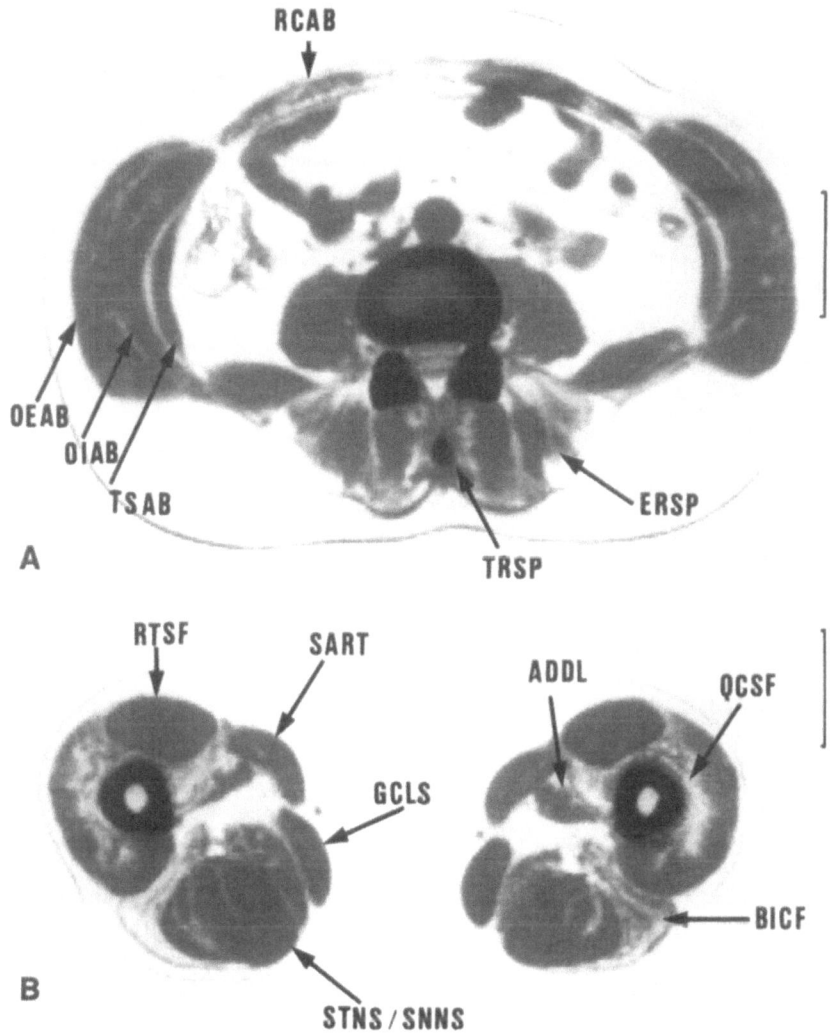

Fig. 6.9. A Compensatory hypertrophy of the m. transversus abdominis (*TSAB*), m. obliquus internus abdominis (*OIAB*) and m. obliquus externus abdominis (*OEAB*) together with atrophy of the mm. recti abdominis (*RCAB*) and the m. transversospinalis (*TRSP*) and m. erector spinae (*ERSP*) in a 53-year-old male with X-linked pseudohypertrophic muscular dystrophy of the Becker type (BECKER and KIENER 1955)

B The thigh muscles of the same patient with compensatory hypertrophy of m. rectus femoris (*RTSF*), m. gracilis (*GCLS*), m. sartorius (*SART*) and m. semitendinosus (*STNS*) and/or semimembranosus (*SNNS*). This complex of hypertrophic muscles can be considered pathognomonic for the disease. Note again the "excavation" of m. quadriceps femoris (*QCSF*), the relative preservation of m. adductor longus (*ADDL*) and the peculiar "onion peel" atrophy of the caput longum of m. biceps femoris (*BICF*). Bar = 5 cm

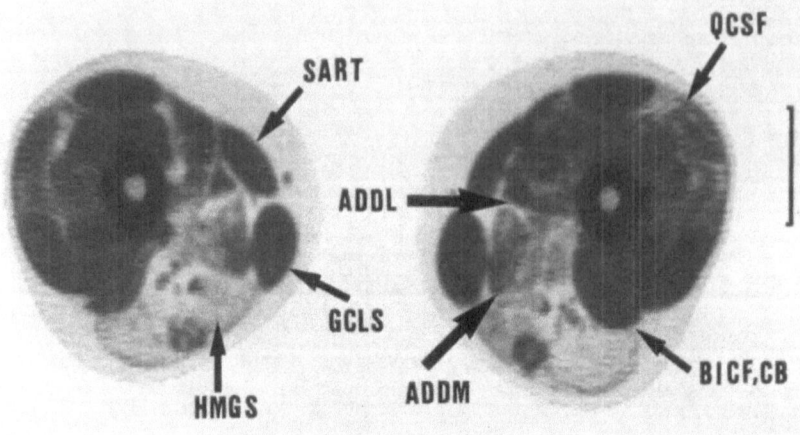

Fig. 6.10. Two totally different patterns of compensatory hypertrophy are found in two brothers with Becker-type muscular dystrophy. The oldest, 44 years old, has lost all hamstring muscles (*HMGS*) and m. adductor magnus (*ADDM*), while m. adductor longus (*ADDL*) is still well preserved, as is the entire m. quadriceps femoris (*QCSF*). Compensatory hypertrophy here is seen in m. sartorius (*SART*), m. gracilis (*GCLS*) and caput breve of m. biceps femoris (*BICF.CB*). This is a rather classical stage in the evolution of the disease. Bar = 5 cm

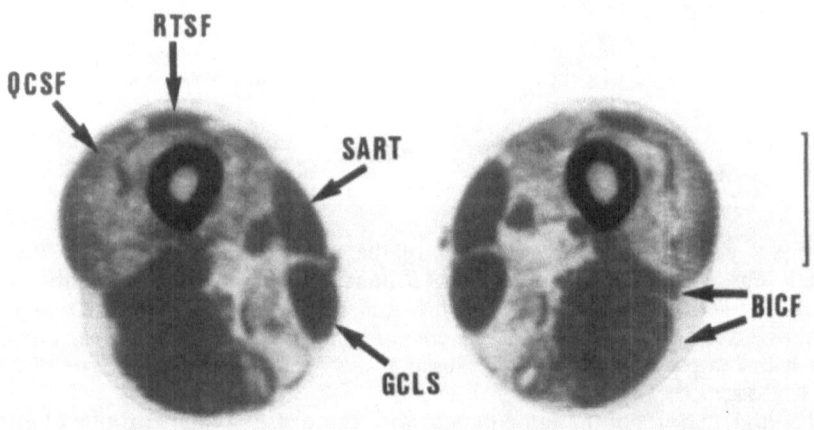

Fig. 6.11. The brother, ten years younger, has severe atrophy of m. quadriceps femoris (*QCSF*) with a remnant of m. rectus femoris (*RTSF*) but hypertrophy of m. sartorius (*SART*), m. gracilis (*GCLS*) and both caput breve and caput longum of m. biceps femoris (*BICF*). This is an aberrant pattern of muscular changes in the same disease. Bar = 5 cm

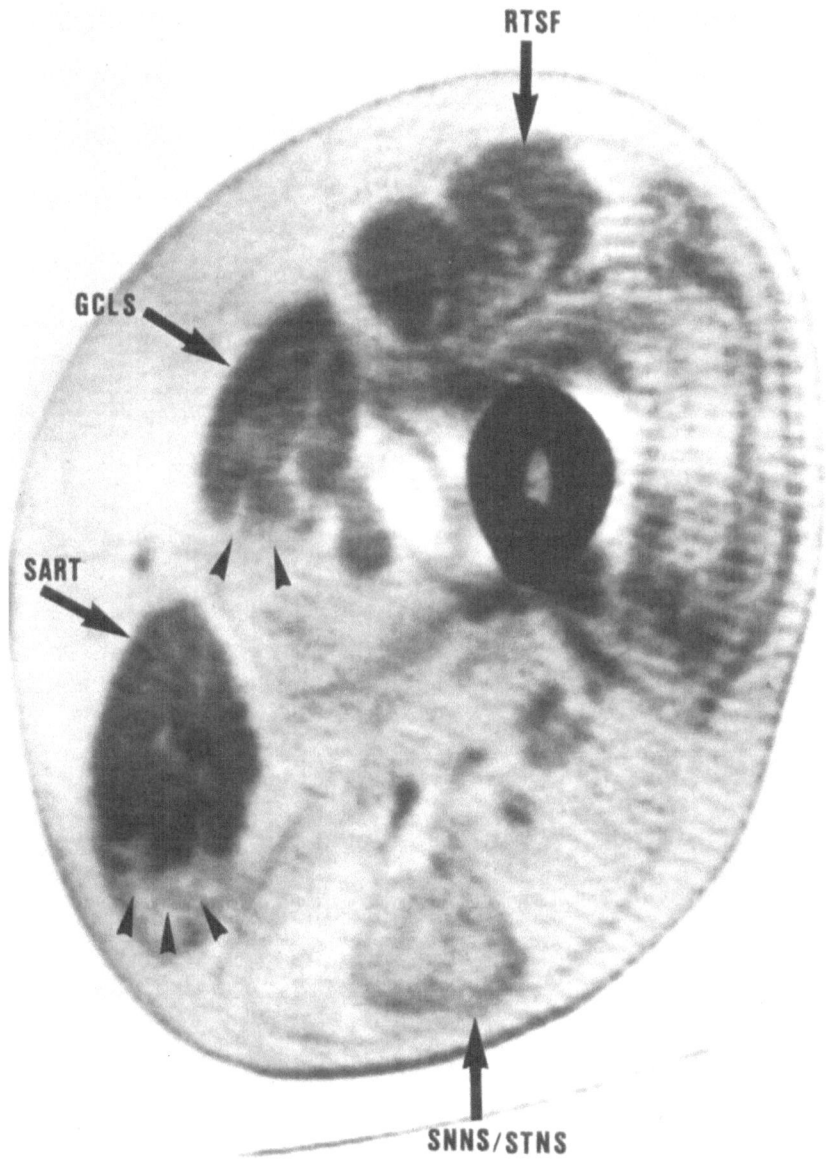

Fig. 6.12. Breakdown (*small arrows*) of the compensatory hypertrophic muscles is the turning point towards end-stage myopathy. This 25-year-old male, also with Becker's disease, shows this breakdown in m. rectus femoris (*RTSF*), m. sartorius (*SART*) and m. gracilis (*GCLS*). The m. semimembranosus (*SNNS*) and m. semitendinosus (*STNS*) have completely disappeared

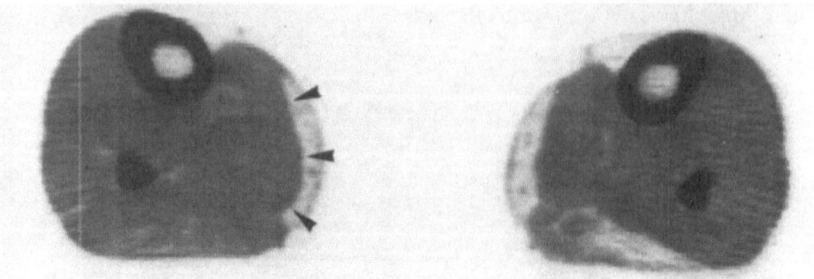

Fig. 6.13

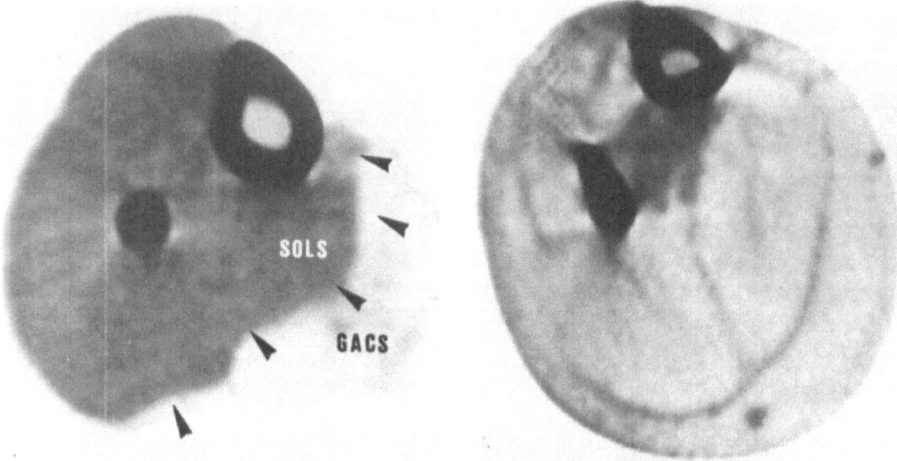

Fig. 6.14

Fig. 6.16

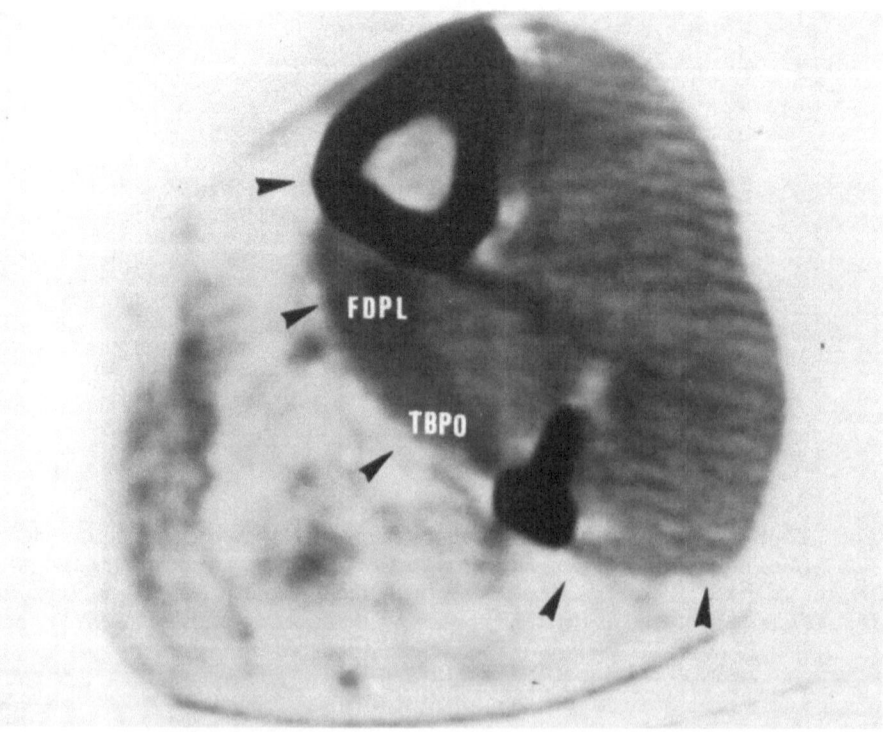

Fig. 6.15

6.1.1.5 End-stage Myopathy

All types of atrophy can finally produce an end-stage in which normal muscle tissue has been almost totally destroyed. The separate lines of evolution of muscular wasting which we have described also lead to two essentially different types of end-stage pictures, however. Cases of spinal muscular atrophy reach an end-stage in which the muscular fasciae have totally disappeared, while the muscles have retreated into tiny islands of ragged muscular tissue. Those cases, on the other hand – mainly of different types of myopathies – which evolve through the filling-up process or with important selectivity and hypertrophy, retain almost normal configurations of structural elements. The panniculus adiposus and the muscle fascia remain in their original position. They are usually devoid of any muscle remnants, and large blood vessels and nerve trunks can still be observed in their original positions. In all cases, the clinical appearance of the patient may, deceptively, fail to suggest any major muscular destruction.

One such case has been thoroughly investigated (Fig. 6.17). A complete autopsy was performed on a large number of muscles. Fat and water content, fat cell volume and radiological density of these muscles were determined (Table 6.1). The fatty acid composition of a series of muscle and fat tissue samples was determined (Table 6.2). Fat and water content were compared with radiological density measurements (Fig. 6.18) and conclusive evidence has been obtained that the low-density material observed in the CT scans is indeed fat tissue with specific histological and biochemical characteristics.

Fig. 6.13. Hypertrophic calf muscles of pathient with Becker muscular dystrophy, already shown in Fig. 6.10 (thigh muscles). Filling-up process is starting under the fascia of both caput mediale and caput laterale (*arrows*) of m. gastrocnemius

Fig. 6.14. Edge (*arrows*) of further filling-up has almost completely passed through m. gastrocnemius (*GACS*) in 38-year-old female with autosomal recessive limb-girdle myopathy of not yet determined aetiology. It has reached m. soleus (*SOLS*), which is still essentially preserved, as is the overall size of the lower leg

Fig. 6.15. Image to Fig. 6.14, almost identical but edge (*arrows*) of filling-up process has reached the deep m. flexor digitorum longus (*FDPL*) and m. tibialis posterior (*TBPO*) in a 53-year-old male with amyotrophic lateral sclerosis

Fig. 6.16. End-stage of filling-up has been reached. Only the deepest muscles are preserved. The lower leg consists of the original size fascia compartments, now lined with fibrotic fasciae. All original muscle compartments are visible and the picture strikingly resembles the line drawing of Fig. 5.17

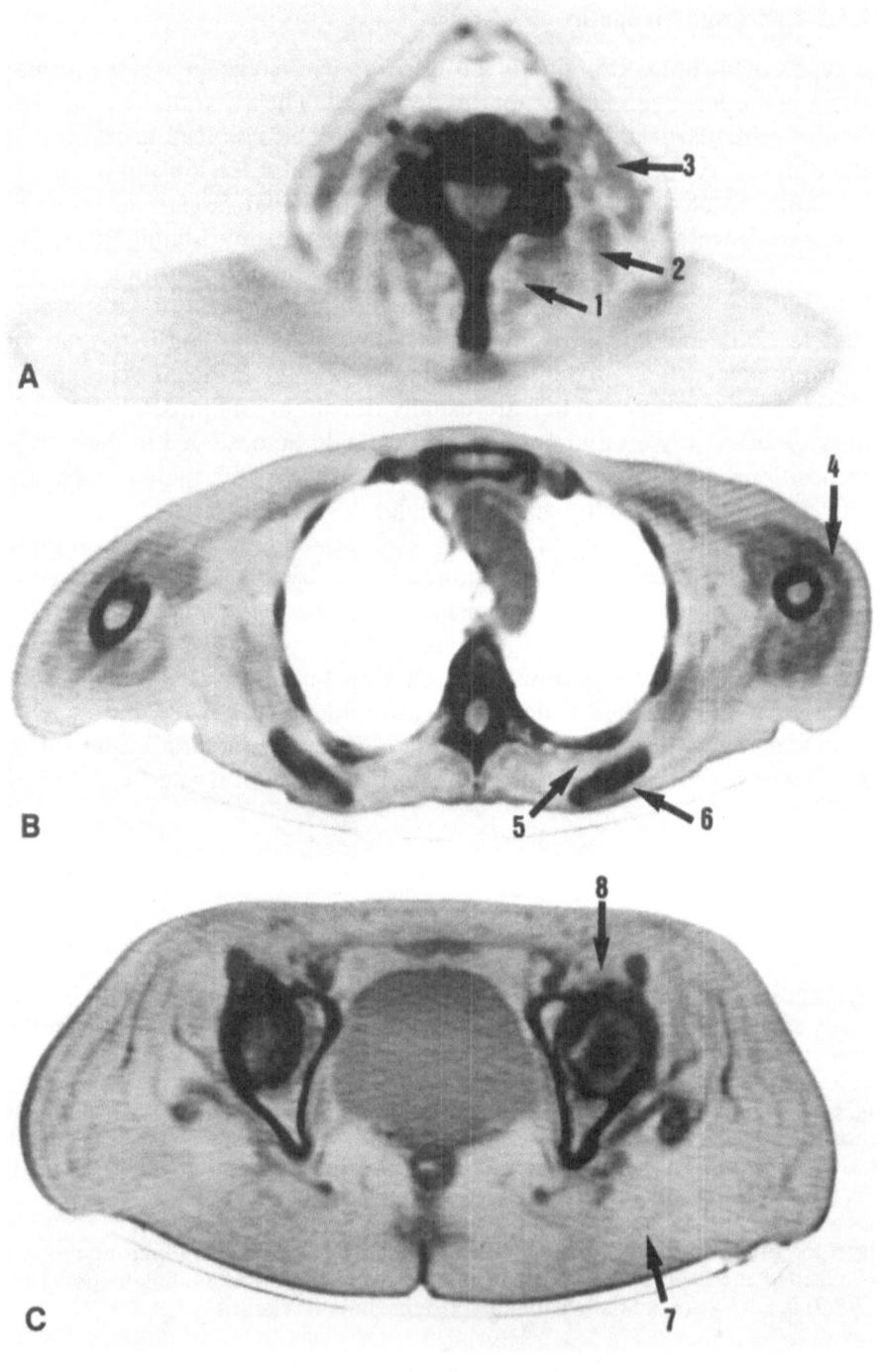

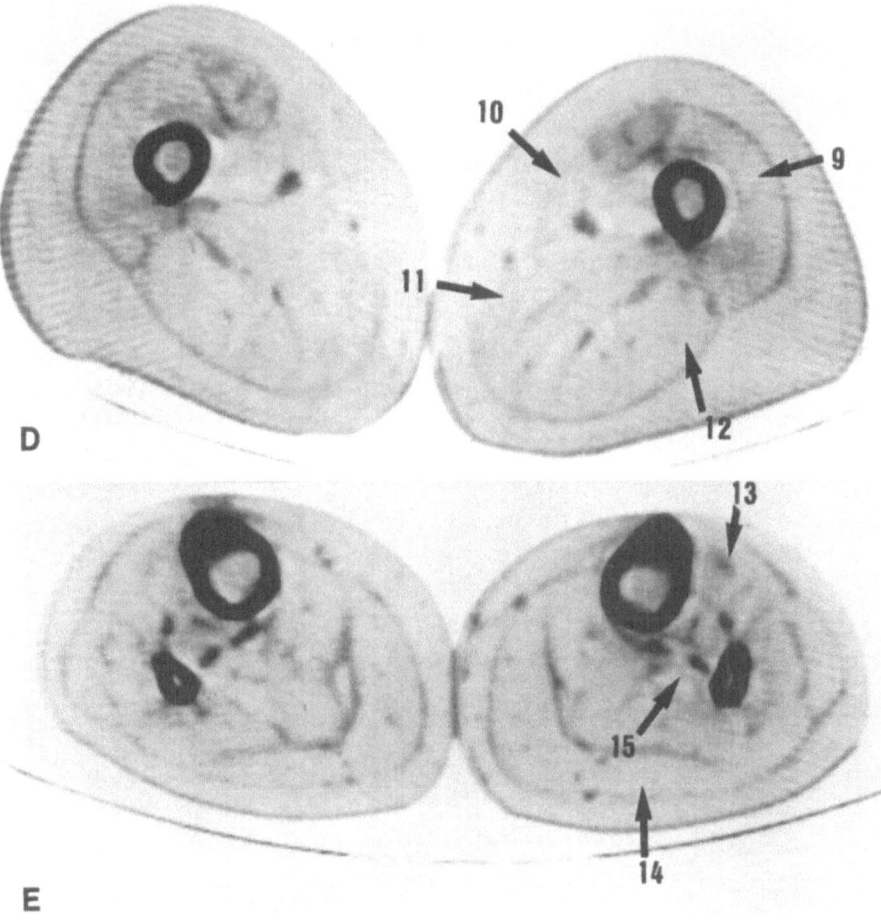

Fig. 6.17 A–E. End-stage myopathy in a 67-year-old female admitted to hospital for terminal care. The diagnosis could not be established, as there were almost no medical documents on a clinical history of at least 20 years of serious symptomatology. Her condition was such that no technical investigations such as biopsy of EMG could be usefully done. The autopsy material did not reveal any particular diagnosis. The patient died 3 weeks after admission. Unfortunately the CT scan taken a few hours before exitus, and on which autopsy sites were selected and density measurements done, could not be used again owing to a technical error and despite much effort by the tape manufacturer. The scans presented were taken on admission and show the approximate biopsy sites and densitometry regions of interest. The numbers on the scans correspond to those in Table 6.1

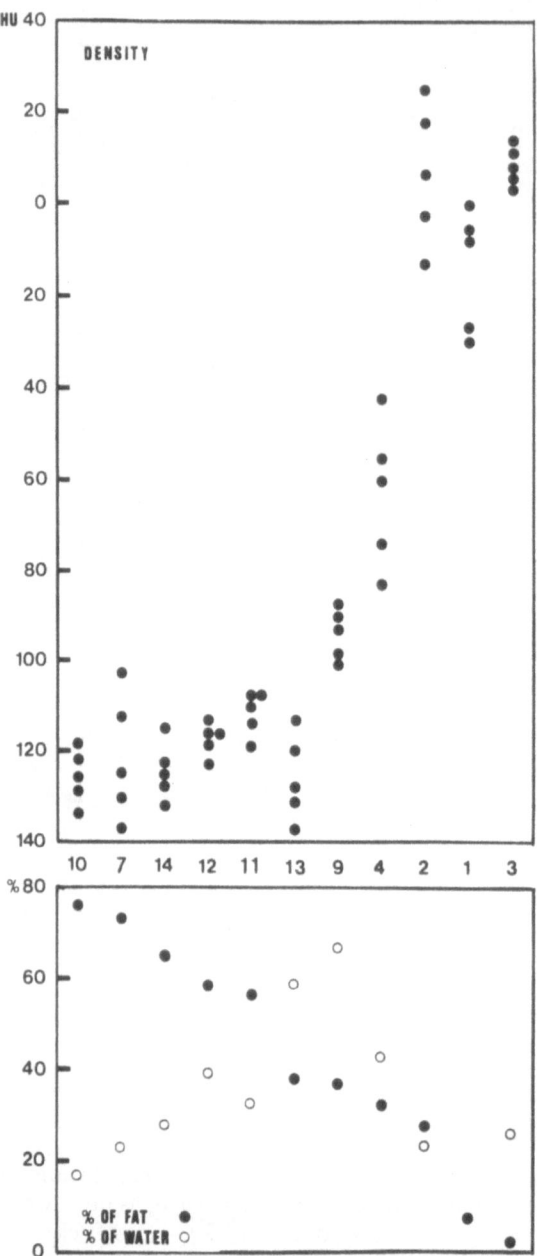

Fig. 6.18. Density measurements in the different muscles. A significant, inversely proportional correlation is observed between density and fat content. All density values are extremely low, and even those muscles with low fat content barely reach the normal density range

Table 6.1. Fat and water content, mean fat cell volume and density measurements of muscle and fat tissue samples

Sample number	Muscle	Fat (%)	Water (%)	Fat cell volume (nl)	Radiological density (HU) (mean ± 2 s.d.)
1	m. erector spinae	9.3	–[b]	0.11	− 13.00 ± 5.81
2	PL. muscle group[a]	29.5	23.5	0.10	+ 38.00 ± 16.99
3	m. sternocleidomastoideus	4.2	25.8	–	+ 9.20 ± 4.11
4	m. deltoideus	34.2	42.6	0.12	− 62.40 ± 27.91
5	m. subscapularis	22.8	38.2	0.13	–
6	m. infraspinatus	31.5	36.9	0.13	–
7	m. gluteus maximus	74.0	22.3	0.15	121.00 ± 54.11
8	m. iliopsoas	39.6	39.0	0.18	–
9	m. vastus lateralis	37.9	67.0	0.16	− 96.80 ± 43.29
10	m. sartorius	79.0	16.6	0.21	− 126.00 ± 56.35
11	m. gracilis	58.1	32.4	0.24	− 108.40 ± 48.48
12	m. biceps femoris	59.1	38.6	0.20	− 117.00 ± 52.32
13	m. tibialis anterior	39.2	59.1	0.32	− 125.40 ± 56.08
14	m. gastrocnemius (caput laterale)	65.0	26.8	0.24	− 124.60 ± 55.72
15	m. tibialis posterior	–	–	–	–
16	m. intercostales (T2-3)	29.5	41.6	0.17	–
17	Diaphragma (pars costalis)	70.7	31.6	0.33	–
18	m. serratus anterior	40.3	49.8	0.10	–
19	m. psoas major	30.5	59.2	0.22	–
20	Subcutaneous fat tissue of abdominal wall	78.1	20.4	0.71	–
21	Perirenal fat tissue	84.4	13.7	0.44	–
22	Omentum fat tissue	81.4	19.2	0.37	–

[a] The posterolateral (PL) muscle group includes m. semispinalis capitis, m. longissimus capitis, m. splenius colli, m. levator scapulae, m. splenius capitis and m. trapezius.
[b] –, not determined

Table 6.2. Fatty acid composition of muscle and fat tissue samples

Sample number	Muscle	14:0[a]	16:0[b]	16:1[c]	18:0[d]	18:1[e]	18:2[f]
4	m. deltoideus	2.0	22.9	9.0	3.6	49.8	12.7
5	m. subscapularis	2.4	24.1	7.2	4.8	47.9	13.6
11	m. gracilis	1.8	20.1	6.5	4.8	52.4	14.4
12	m. biceps femoris	1.6	21.8	6.8	4.5	52.8	12.4
17	Diaphragma (pars costalis)	3.0	21.1	9.2	4.0	48.9	13.8
20	Subcutaneous fat of abdominal wall	2.0	19.6	7.2	3.1	53.4	14.7
21	Perirenal fat tissue	2.6	23.8	6.4	4.8	48.0	14.4
22	Omentum fat tissue	2.4	21.7	10.4	3.9	48.4	13.2

[a] 14:0, myristic acid
[b] 16:0, palmitic acid
[c] 16:1, palmitoleic acid
[d] 18:0, stearic acid
[e] 18:1, oleic acid
[f] 18:2, linoleic acid

6.1.1.6 The Most Resistant Muscles

In all cases of end-stage myopathy the most resistant muscles were found to be the neck muscles and the deepest muscles in the lower legs, more specifically the m. tibialis posterior and the m. flexor digitorum longus (Fig. 6.19).

6.1.2 Muscular Atrophy as a Selective Process

Numerous CT scan pictures of neuromuscular diseases clearly demonstrate that atrophy of skeletal muscles tends to be remarkably selective. This selectivity was found to be present on three levels.

6.1.2.1 Inter-group Selectivity

The long-known clinical selectivity between proximal and distal muscles is clearly visible in CT scans and can now be amply documented and used clinically. Most neuromuscular diseases studied so far do start as proximal limb-girdle diseases, particularly with the pelvic and thigh muscles. This is clearly different from peripheral neuropathies and some myopathies in which distal muscles are the first to be affected. Another example is the distinction between atrophy of extensor and flexor muscle groups (Figs. 6.20, 6.21).

6.1.2.2 Inter-muscular Selectivity

On each level of the standard examination procedure some individual muscles show significant degrees of atrophy while others seem to be very resistant to any form of atrophy. This type of selectivity is especially striking for a number of muscles, particularly in the lower extremities. These muscles all seem to have the common characteristics of a stretched-out, fusiform profile. Primary examples are the m. gracilis and the m. sartorius, which may remain unaffected even in cases of severe atrophy of the thigh muscles of any aetiology. This resistance of fusiform muscles is, however, not absolute; rarely, they are selectively atrophic as well.

6.1.2.3 Intra-muscular Selectivity

Selectivity of muscular atrophy is also found in parts of compound muscles such as the m. quadriceps femoris, the m. triceps surae (m. gastrocnemius

---

Fig. 6.20. Inter-group selectivity in a 36-year-old male with chronic polymyositis. The extensor group, here mainly the m. quadriceps femoris (*QCSF*), is well preserved except for the m. rectus femoris (*RTSF*). The groups of the knee flexors, of the hamstrings (*HMGS*) and of the adductores (*ADDS*) are severely atrophic. M. sartorius (*SART*) and m. gracilis (*GCLS*) are well preserved

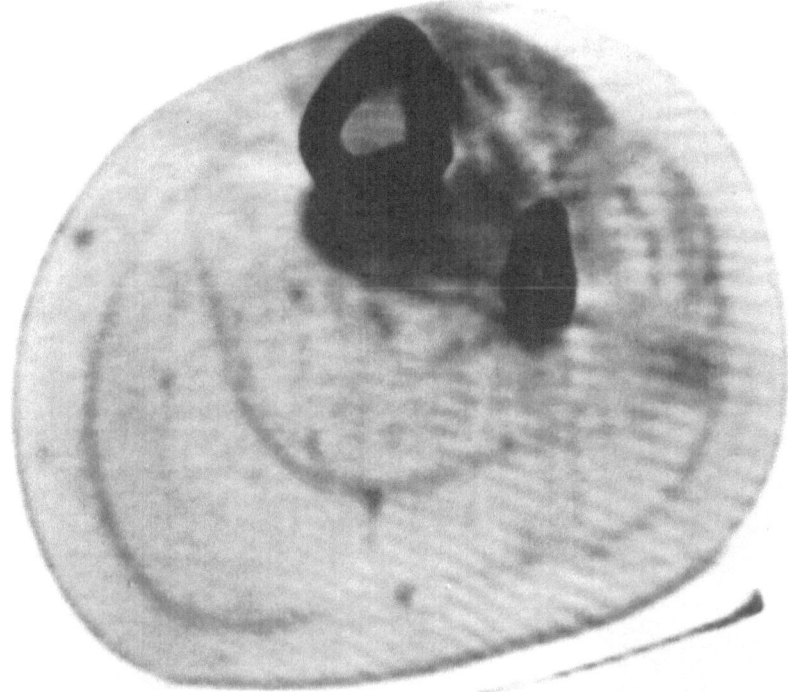

Fig. 6.19. End-stage of a limb-girdle muscular dystrophy in a 33-year-old female. Only the m. flexor digitorum longus and m. tibialis posterior are still present

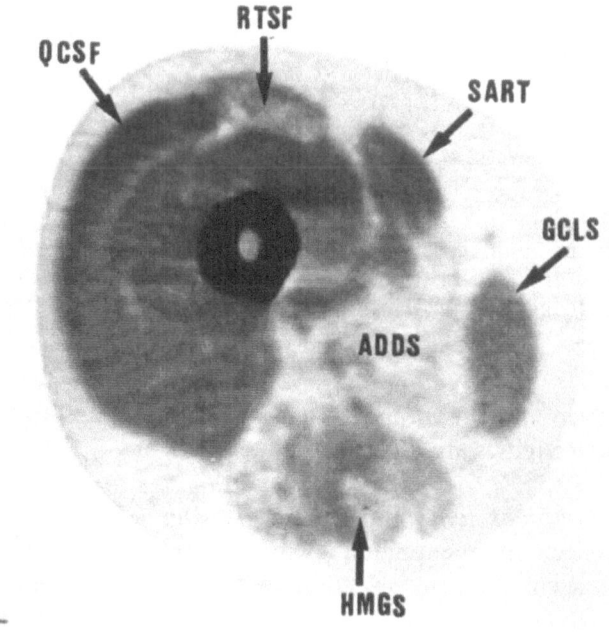

Fig. 6.20

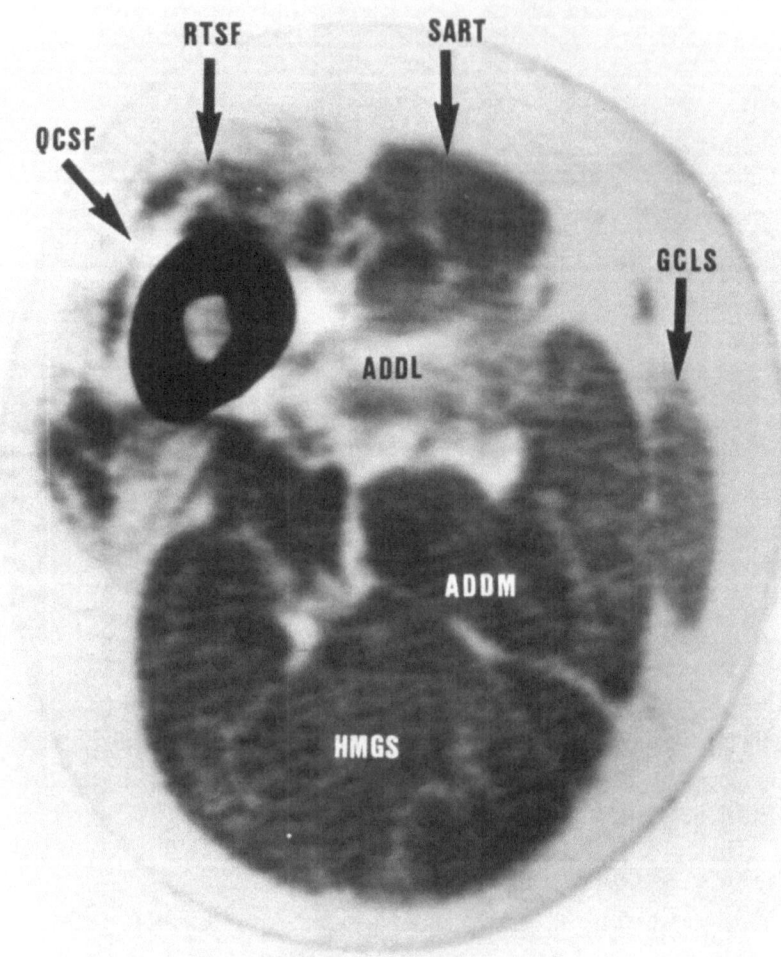

Fig. 6.21. Inter-group selectivity but in a reverse pattern to that of Fig. 6.20. This 53-year-old patient with amyotrophic lateral sclerosis has selective atrophy of the extensor group – in this case the complete m. quadriceps femoris (*QCSF*), including m. rectus femoris (*RTSF*) – and also of the m. adductor longus (*ADDL*), while m. adductor magnus (*ADDM*), the hamstrings (*HMGS*), m. sartorius (*SART*) and m. gracilis (*GCLS*) are better preserved

and m. soleus) and the m. biceps femoris. In Fig. 6.22 most of these intra-muscular selectivities are illustrated in one patient.

The m. quadriceps femoris is perhaps the most striking example of the muscular selectivity phenomenon, with two different aspects.

First, it seems that the selectivity of atrophy which applies to the fusiform m. gracilis and m. sartorius also applies to the m. rectus femoris,

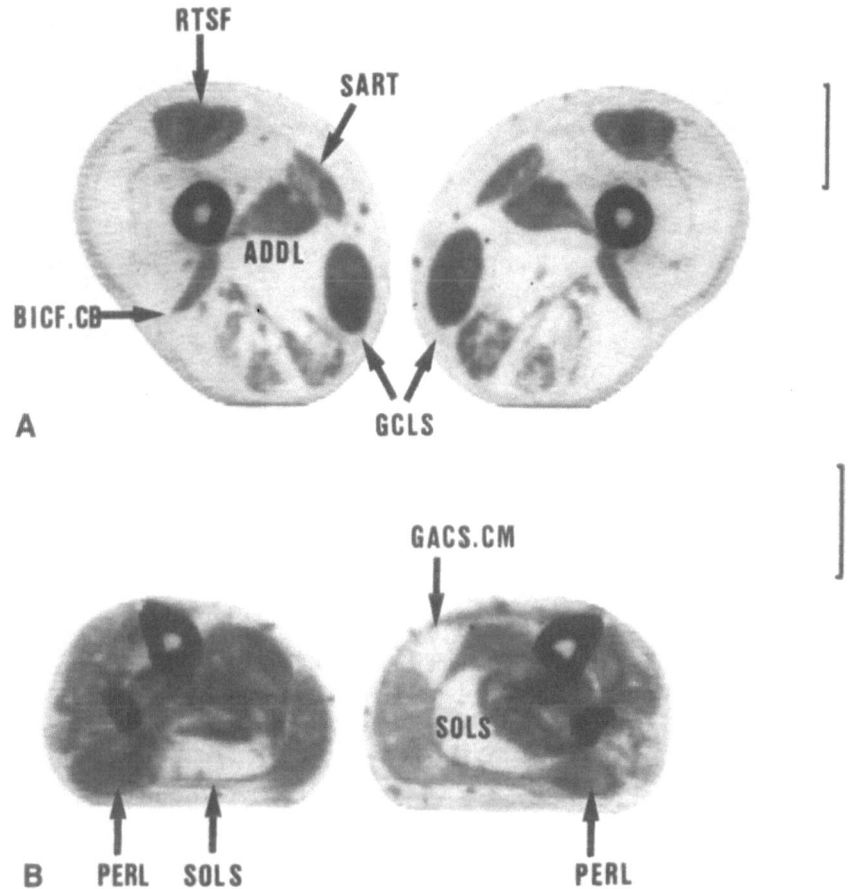

Fig. 6.22. A Scan of a 46-year-old male with a peculiar polysaccharide-accumulation myopathy, showing most of the fusiform muscles in the thigh which are usually preserved in different myopathies. They are the m. rectus femoris (*RTSF*), the m. sartorius (*SART*), the m. gracilis (*GCLS*), the m. biceps femoris, caput breve (*BICF.CB*) and here also the m. adductor longus (*ADDL*). Bar = 5 cm
B Lower leg muscles of same patient show "punched out" m. soleus (*SOLS*) and atrophy of one part of m. gastrocnemius, caput mediale, on the right side (*GACS.CM*). Both sides show hypertrophy of m. peroneus longus (*PERL*)

which represents the fusiform part of the m. quadriceps. Many examples can be found in which this part of the m. quadriceps is selectively spared; this can also be seen in Fig. 6.22. In this particular case, by putting an SFEMG into the m. rectus femoris under CT control, we obtained electrophysical evidence that we were not simply looking at remnants of the original muscle, but that an active regenerative process was taking place in this muscle (see Table 8.3), enabling the patient to stand and walk without any aid.

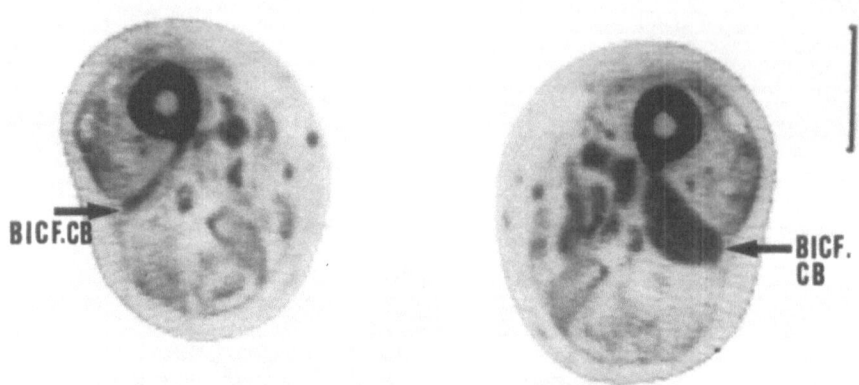

Fig. 6.23. Extreme example of selectivity within the m. biceps femoris in a 44-year-old patient with spinal muscular atrophy of the Kugelberg-Welander type. Only caput breve (*BICF.CB*) is preserved and hypertrophic on the right side, but this patient is walking independently with knee bracing. Bar = 5 cm

Secondly, some of the scans already shown lead us to conclude that in certain diseases, e.g. myotonic dystrophy, atrophy of the m. quadriceps femoris follows a very definite sequence: it seems to originate in the m. vastus intermedius, spreading centrifugally towards the m. vastus lateralis and m. vastus medialis and finally towards the m. rectus femoris. In some cases the m. vastus lateralis seems literally "excavated", leaving only a shell of muscle tissue at the periphery. A striking example is found in Fig. 7.20.

The m. triceps surae. A very similar selection process can be found in another compound muscle, the m. triceps surae. In many cases the first part of this muscle complex to be affected is the m. soleus, while the m. gastrocnemius remains well preserved. In some diseases, this process seems to be accelerated so that the m. soleus is almost selectively "punched out" (Fig. 6.22 B). When the latter is finally also affected, it is usually the caput mediale which is affected first while the caput laterale remains preserved until late in the disease.

The m. biceps femoris consists of a fusiform caput breve and a more compact caput longum. Here again, the fusiform part is the last to disappear and is frequently seen to be hypertrophic (Fig. 6.23).

Several hypotheses can be submitted to explain selective atrophy and/or hypertrophy of muscles. Among the possible causes are either the blood supply or the innervation pattern; for instance, caput breve and caput longum of m. biceps femoris are innervated by different nerves. The hypothesis that the selectivity of muscular atrophy is based on the diversity in fibre-type composition could also be of relevance; for example, a centrifugal gradient of atrophy such as seen in the m. quadriceps could be explained if the different fibre types are so arranged. At present, however, none of these hypotheses can be proven responsible for the observed phenomena. Most muscles involved in a selective atrophic process cannot be attributed to either a particular neurogenic or vascular territory, nor do the presently known fibre-type patterns of muscles exhibit any particular gradient in compound muscles. One of the major problems in evaluating this selectivity of atrophy is the enormous plasticity of skeletal muscle (PETTE 1980) and the probably continuous regenerative muscular activity. The residual muscles seen in CT scans of progressive neuromuscular disease are probably not merely remnants of the original muscle, but continuously remodeled structures with little or no resemblance to the original muscle.

6.2 Muscular Hypertrophy

Muscular hypertrophy can be defined as an increase in muscular volume above the normal limits for a particular muscle. It can be easily observed on CT scans of the skeletal muscular system and can be translated into numerical data by measuring the surface area of the transversely cut muscle by means of built-in programs. Once the normal size of the same muscle at the same CT scan level is known, the diagnosis of muscular hypertrophy can be established and its degree fairly accurately measured.

True muscular hypertrophy (i.e. non-neoplastic), can be produced by three basic mechanisms. Either the volume of the muscle cells remains unchanged but the number increases or the number remains stable while the volume increases, or both mechanisms are activated at the same time. These underlying mechanisms cannot be differentiated on CT scans; only histopathological techniques can verify them. There are, however, other conditions which result in an increase in the volume of a muscle, for instance the infiltration of the muscle by other types of cells, such as fat cells. This phenomenon is called pseudohypertrophy and can easily be seen on CT scans. Examples both of true muscular hypertrophy and of pseudohypertrophy will be presented in this chapter.

6.2.1 Muscular Hypertrophy of Athletes as a Normal Variant

Perhaps the best-known example of muscular hypertrophy is the increase in muscle volume which occurs when healthy muscles are subjected to increased workloads, owing either to the normal occupation of the subject or to planned training programs of athletes. This type of hypertrophy can be considered a variant of normal in which the upper limits of normal are physiologically extended. Under training conditions the volume of the muscles being trained is indeed increased, but other significant events are also observed, such as a decrease in interstitial tissue and in panniculus adiposus around the muscles, producing a dense packing of muscles in which the individual muscular boundaries are no longer visible. CT scanning of athletes could therefore provide a rather accurate assessment of the effectiveness of their training.

6.2.2 Myotonic Disorders and Denervation Hypertrophy

Muscular hypertrophy is also frequently observed in pathological conditions, both in myopathies, in which the biochemical defect is thought to be in the muscle itself, and in chronic neurogenic diseases, in which there is denervation hypersensitivity of the muscles. The best-known example of a group of myopathies in which hypertrophy has been demonstrated is the myotonic diseases in particular myotonia congenita, in which the continuous contractions of the muscles are thought to be responsible for the muscular hypertrophy. Muscular hypertrophy is also found in chronic neurogenic conditions in which the denervation causes a hypersensitivity of the muscles to stimulation, resulting in denervation hypertrophy. In both conditions the hypertrophy is rather generalized with very little atrophy present.

6.2.3 Compensatory Hypertrophy

Compensatory hypertrophy occurs in situations in which selective atrophy occurs in one or more muscles or parts of muscle of a synergistic functional group, forcing the remaining muscles or parts of muscle to carry the additional work-load of the atrophic muscles. They undergo what is usually called compensatory hypertrophy, which has already been described.

6.2.4 Hypertrophy and Pseudohypertrophy of m. triceps surae

Muscular hypertrophy and pseudohypertrophy are perhaps best known in the X-linked muscular dystrophies, and more particularly in Duchenne muscular dystrophy (DMD) and Becker muscular dystrophy (BMD). It has been demonstrated by means of CT scanning (BULCKE et al. 1981) that in these diseases a transition process takes place from true hypertrophy at the onset of the disease (Fig. 6.24) to pseudohypertrophy in which muscular atrophy is compensated by fat tissue infiltration (Fig. 6.25), finally leading to complete atrophy of all muscles but with continued preservation of the original hypertrophic aspect of the lower leg.

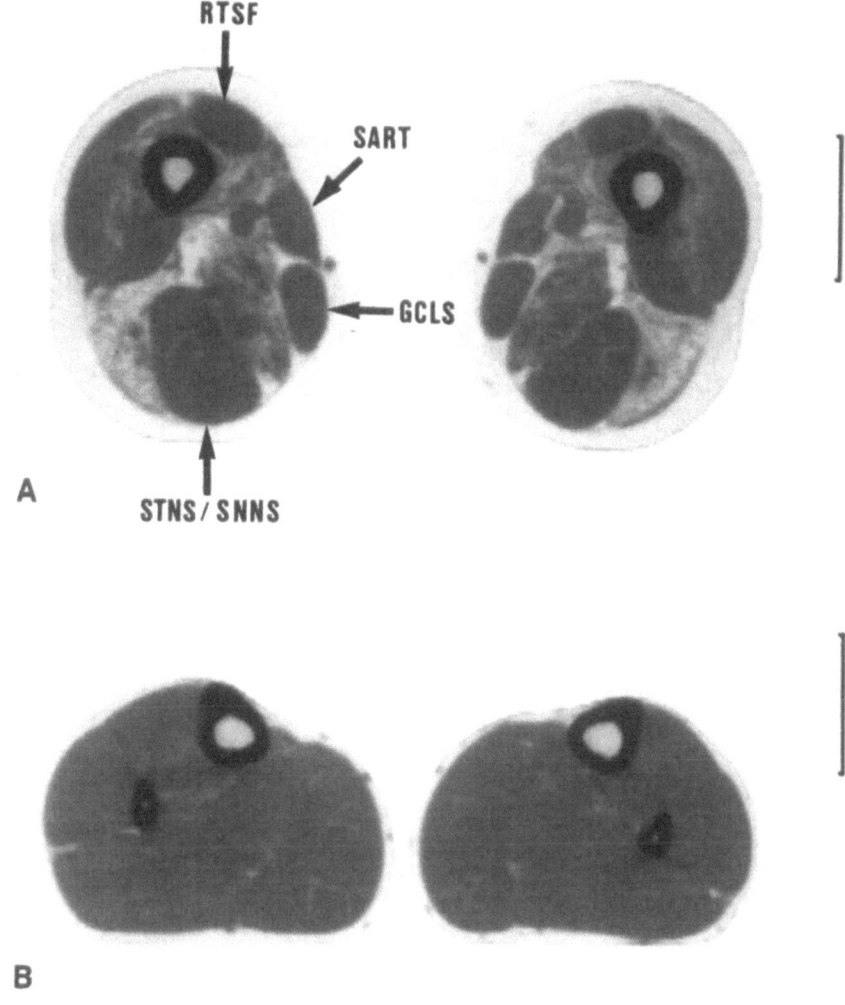

Fig. 6.24 A, B. Initial stage of Becker muscular dystrophy in a 24-year-old patient. **A** The thigh muscles show the first characteristic step in the evolution of this disease with hypertrophy of m. rectus femoris (*RTSF*), m. sartoirus (*SART*), m. gracilis (*GCLS*) and the m. semitendinosus (*STNS*) and semimembranosus (*SNNS*). **B** The lower leg muscles are even larger in size than the thigh muscles (*linear index* represents 5 cm) but they are dense and strong. Bar = 5 cm

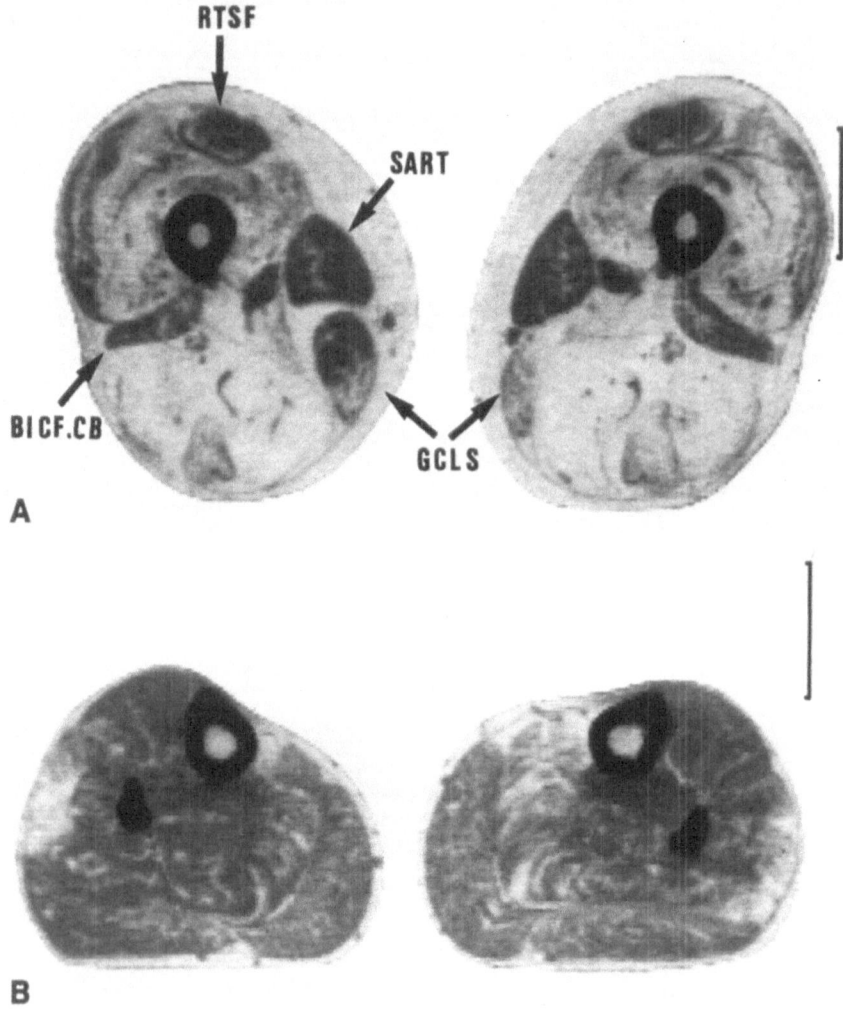

Fig. 6.25 A, B. Thirty-year-old patient with same disease as shown in Fig. 6.24. **A** The thigh muscle shave passed the stage of compensatory hypertrophy. The once hypertrophic muscles (m. rectus femoris (*RTSF*), m. sartorius (*SART*), m. gracilis (*GCLS*) and m. biceps femoris, caput breve (*BICF.CB*)) now undergo in turn a process of progessive muscular wasting. **B** The lower leg muscles are still almost as large as the thigh muscles, but are heavily infiltrated by fat in a "whirlwind" pattern. This is "pseudohypertrophy". Bar = 5 cm

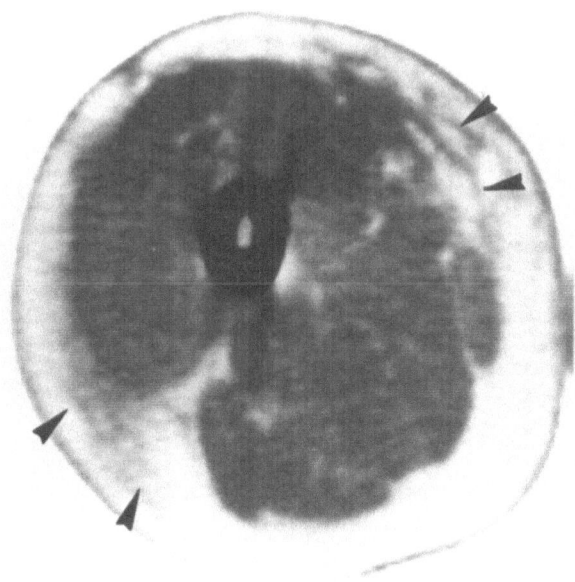

Fig. 6.26. Thigh muscles of a 25-year-old female with a fibrosing myopathy due to years of pentazocine abuse. Subcutaneous shells of fibrosis (*arrows*) are seen, and were probably responsible for the wood-like consistency of the limbs, which were fixed in severe ankyloses at knee and elbow joints

6.3 Muscular Hypotrophy

Although, as has been shown, muscular atrophy does not necessarily lead to muscular hypotrophy, at least not when the volume of different types of tissue within the original fascia is considered, many diseases do finally lead to a diminished muscular volume which can then also become clinically visible. It must be stressed, however, that the two phenomena are independent of each other, and that measuring the size of a muscle or a group of muscles does not necessarily give any information about its trophic condition.

6.4 Fibrosis of Muscular and Subcutaneous Tissues

Infiltration of muscle by fibrotic tissue is, as far as could be ascertained by means of CT scanning of a large series of various neuromuscular diseases, a rather rare event and certainly not of the same extent as infiltration by fat tissue. A number of examples were found in which strands of fibrotic tissue

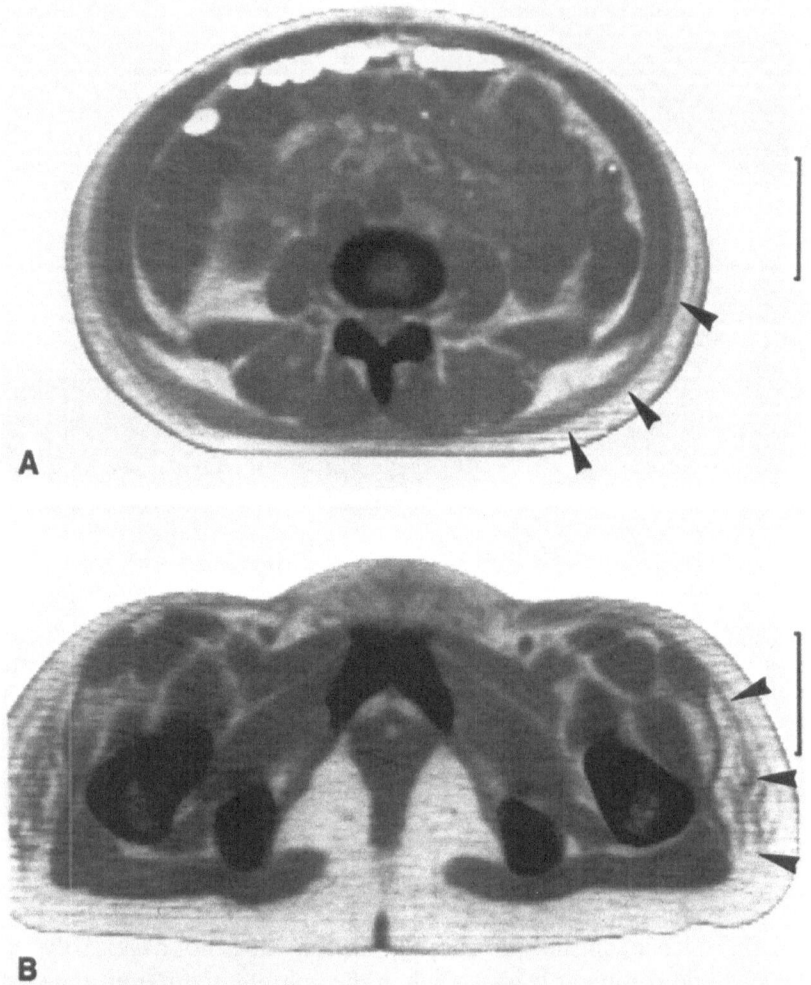

Fig. 6.27 A, B. Abdominal and spinal muscular scans of a 21-year-old female admitted to the emergency department in cardiac arrest with a hyperacute alcoholic cardio-rhabdomyolysis. The extremely high myoglobin levels in serum could not be accurately measured by radio-immunoassay, but the patient lost approximately 25 g myoglobin in the urine on the day of admission, during which she had three cardiac arrests. Myoglobin is seen **A** in the subcutaneous fat against the subcutaneous fascia with the patient in the supine position (*arrows*) and **B** in the form of streaks "running" downwards in the pelvic subcutaneous fat (*arrows*). Bar = 5 cm

could be observed in muscular and subcutaneous tissues. In most of these cases the fibrosis seemed to proceed independently of muscle atrophy and could be attributed to specific causes such as long-standing drug abuse (Fig. 6.26). It could be, however, that in the cases where it was not observed fibrosis was present either as a variable number of small reticular fibrils in

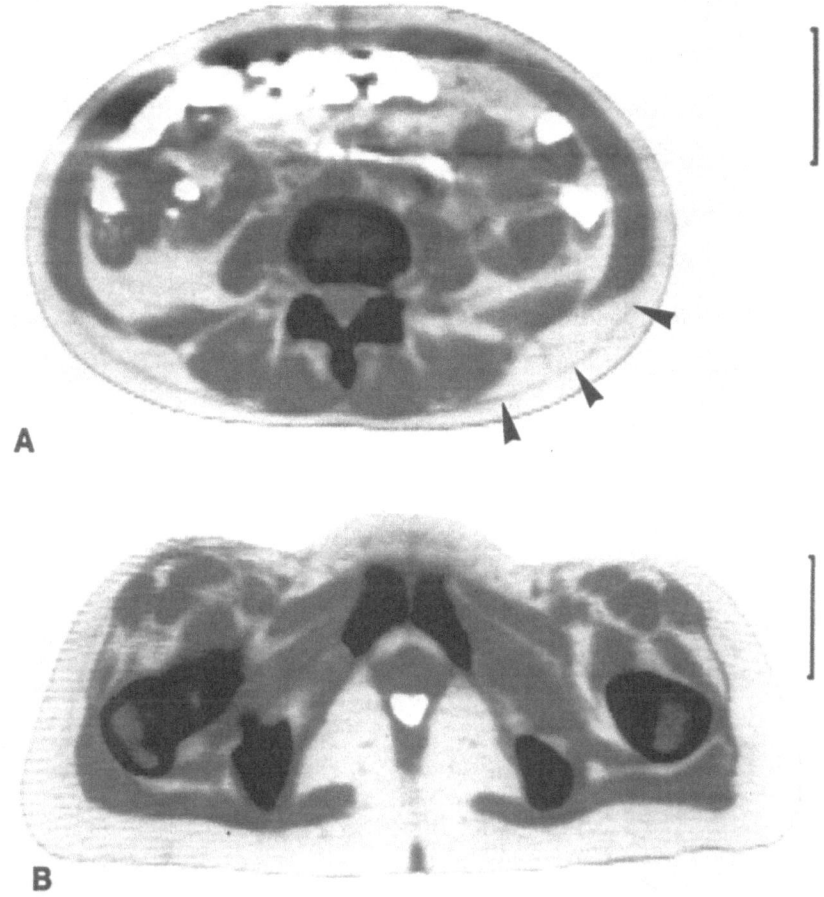

Fig. 6.28 A, B. Same levels of same patient exactly 3 weeks later. All biochemical parameters have returned to normal. The subcutaneous myoglobin has disappeared but the fascia against which it was positioned is now clearly visible (*arrows*). The pelvic muscles and all others have become hypotrophic. The patient has recovered completely, so far without complications such as fibrosis. Bar = 5 cm

the endomysium, which would be difficult to see, or as an increase in collagen deposit in thickened perimysia and aponeuroses which would be difficult to measure with the CT scanning technique. Fibrosis of the muscular fasciae does occur, however, and has been observed many times (Figs. 6.16, 6.17 D, E, 6.19).

In the differential diagnosis of subcutaneous fibrosis, attention must be drawn to the possibility of reversible infiltration of subcutaneous tissue by muscular-breakdown products such as myoglobin (Figs. 6.27, 6.28) and the existence of fascia-type separations within subcutaneous tissue which are not clearly described in standard anatomy textbooks.

7 Patterns of Muscular Lesions in Several Myopathies

It is obvious that within the framework of this monograph only a limited number of cases can be presented. The selection of scans in this chapter was made on the following basis. First of all, we were limited to the cases of neuromuscular diseases which were admitted to our hospital during the period after the introduction of CT scanning as a routine procedure in the investigation of myopathies. This included a large group of patients with myotonic dystrophy which, because of its dominant inheritance, represents statistically a larger group in any hospital where myopathies are investigated. Secondly, during the same period a number of specific investigative projects were going on, leading to re-admission and more intensive follow-up in the out-patient department of diagnoses which are otherwise not so frequently seen, such as X-linked pseudohypertrophic muscular dystrophy of the Becker type. These two factors led to relatively more extensive sections on these two diseases. Particularly for myotonic dystrophy, this also gave us the opportunity to demonstrate how, when enough scans are available of patients of different ages with the same disease, the natural course of the disease can probably be reconstructed quite accurately. A third and perhaps most decisive factor in selecting our cases was of course the importance of the morphological changes. This is why relatively little attention is given to such a frequently occuring diagnosis as myasthenia gravis in which CT abnormalities are of minor importance.

As we have already described, myopathies can be defined as diseases of the lower motor units. We will therefore successively describe muscular lesions in spinal muscular atrophies, in peripheral neuropathies, in myasthenia gravis and in myopathies in the strict sense. The last category will be more extensively reviewed.

The large majority of diagnoses were made by means of a multidisciplinary investigation during hospital admission as described in Chap. 2, and conform to generally accepted criteria. They are named as much as possible according to the nomenclature and classification proposed by the World Federation of Neurology (1974) and adapted by WALTON (1981).

7.1 Spinal Muscular Atrophies (s.m.a.)

As described in Chap. 2, s.m.a. is the name given to a number of disorders of the motor neurons in brain stem nuclei and in the anterior horn of the spinal cord. In the context of myopathies, the name is usually reserved for the genetically determined diseases of motor neurons. Developmental abnormalities, such as agenesis of cranial nerve nuclei (Moebius' syndrome), destruction or compression of anterior horn cells due to trauma, toxins such as those of *Clostridium tetani*, infections, malignant diseases and metabolic disorders acting on the motor neurons may all produce muscular wasting, usually designated as amyotrophy, very similar to that seen in s.m.a.

We will restrict our description of s.m.a. to cases of the chronic proximal form of the type described by WOHLFART et al. (1955) and by KUGELBERG and WELANDER (1956). They described an autosomal recessive disease with a limb-girdle weakness syndrome, beginning mainly in the pelvic muscles with gait disturbances. Mean age of onset is around adolescence and the course is chronic and very slowly progressive. The distal muscles and the proximal shoulder muscles are usually affected late in the disease, and the life expectancy can be normal. That this disease is of motor neuron origin is confirmed by fasciculations with motor neuron characteristics, which can be seen clinically or on EMG, and by muscle biopsy with typical neurogenic changes such as type-grouping of fibres.

A selection was made from 26 CT scans of 17 patients with different forms of spinal muscular atrophy. The youngest patient was 4 years old, the oldest was 62 at the time of scanning. From these scans we tried to reconstruct the evolution of chronic anterior horn cell disease as it might have occurred in each patient. We have, however, no proof of such an evolution, as our longest follow-up in this group is of one individual patient for only 42 months.

The line of progression which seems to be followed corresponds almost completely with the first pathway of muscular wasting described in Fig. 6.1. It starts with patches of low-density tissue appearing in the muscles whose motor neurons are affected. The main characteristic of these patches is that they are initially very small, very sharp and very diffusely spread all over the surface of the muscles. The initial stage, in which clinically the first fas-

---

Fig. 7.1 A–C. Twenty-year-old female with onset of progressive spinal muscular atrophy of the Kugelberg-Welander type. The disease at the different levels is still in the stage of infiltration by small patches of low-density tissue, diffusely in all muscles, but the moth-eaten aspect is best seen in **C** (*arrows*) because of the enlargement of the picture. In **A** the m. obturatorius internus (*OBIN*) on the left side is totally atrophic. Bar = 5 cm

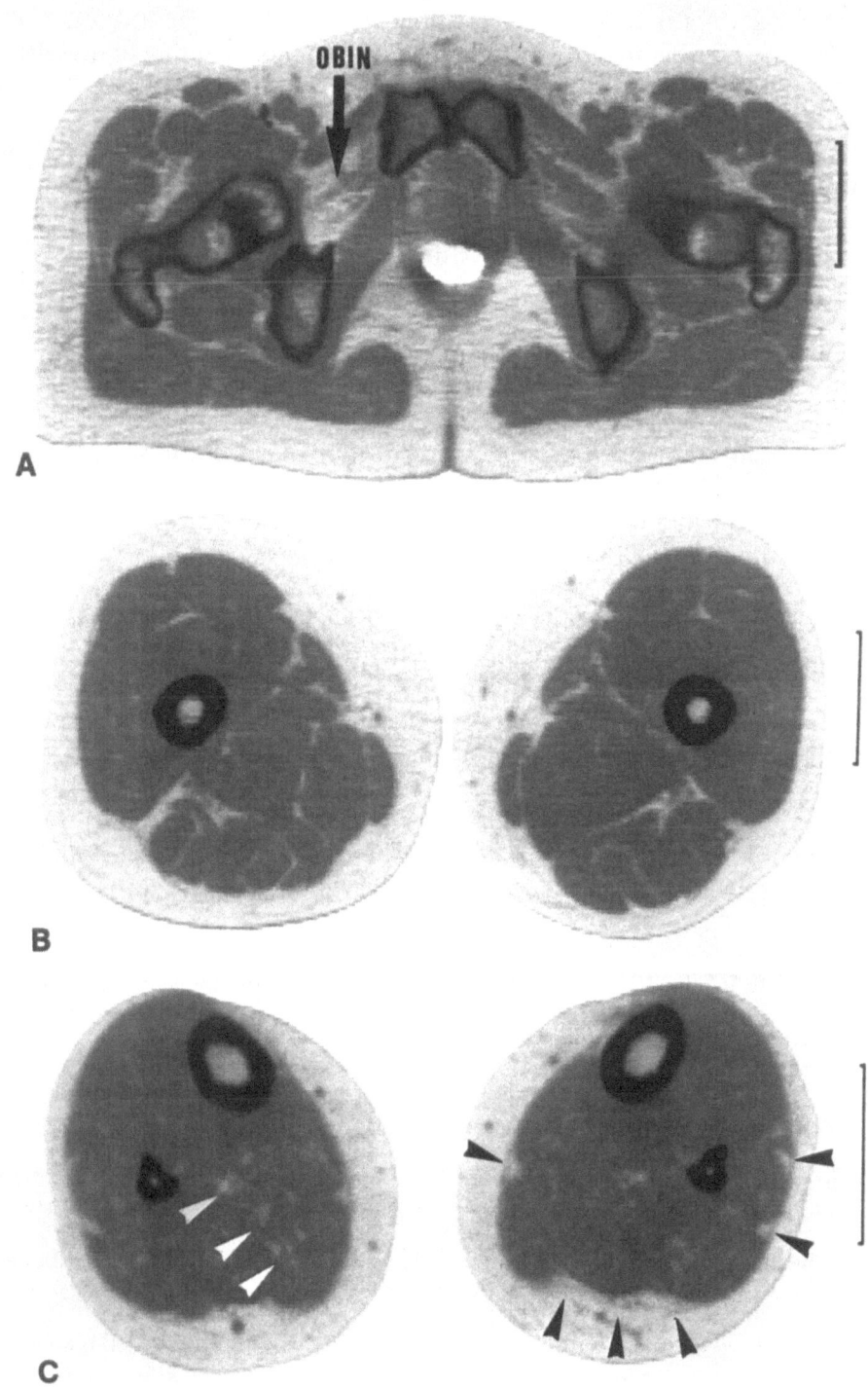

Fig. 7.1 A–C

ciculations appear, is therefore very difficult to reproduce photographically. It is quite possible that this pattern is related to the scattering of muscle fibres of one motor neuron over a certain area of muscle, usually called the motor unit territory.

As the disease progresses the patches become larger – perhaps due to atrophy of smaller and larger type groups which are being formed from the onset of the disease owing to collateral sprouting of motor units not yet affected – and progressively increase their fibre density. This stage is seen in Fig. 7.1 C.

As the disease progresses the muscles acquire an increasingly ragged outline, and at the same time seem to retract from their most distal boundaries towards the proximal insertions on the skeletal elements. The muscles seem to progressively submerge into the panniculus adiposus (Fig. 7.2). This is a first and most pathognomonic feature of s.m.a. at this stage. The distance between the muscular fascia and the skin increases progressively, which is probably the reason why fasciculations become less visible as the disease progresses, although there is no reason to believe that they diminish in intensity. In many other myopathies, in contrast to the s.m.a., the muscles and their fasciae remain in their original positions but either break down in situ or are filled up with mesenchymal elements.

During the centripetal involution of the muscular tissue a second pathognomonic feature becomes visible, the ragged disintegration of the muscular tissues without selectivity or compensatory hypertrophy (Figs. 7.3–7.5).

As do all other neuromuscular disases, spinal muscular atrophies finally evolve towards an end-stage which is characterized by ragged islands of muscular tissue within a large mass of panniculus adiposus (Fig. 7.6).

Fig. 7.2. When the disease progresses, as in this 50-year-old female, the muscles acquire an increasingly ragged outline, without selectivity or compensatory hypertrophy. At the same time the muscles seem to retract from their most distal boundaries towards the proximal insertions on the skeletal elements. They seem to "submerge" into the panniculus adiposus. These aspects can be considered pathognomonic for spinal muscular atrophies

Fig. 7.3. This 42-year-old patient with chronic spinal muscular atrophy further illustrates the "withdrawal" of the muscular tissue towards the proximal muscular insertions, demonstrating at the same time another pathognomonic feature, the "ragged" breakdown of the muscles illustrated in both mm. glutei maximi (*GLMX*) and particularly in the prime movers of the hip (*arrows*)

Fig. 7.4. The way muscles disintegrate in spinal muscular atrophy is well illustrated in this scan of a 29-year-old female. Paricularly at the level of the mm. adductores (*ADDS*) and the hamstrings (*HMGS*) the muscles become "cloudy" and their outlines very ill defined

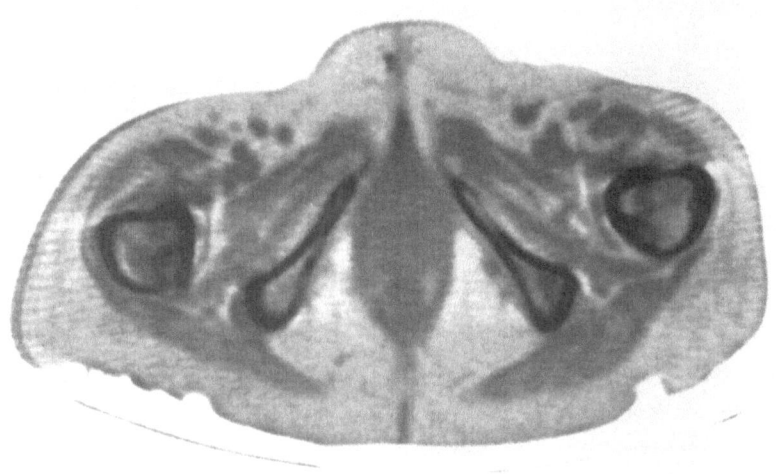

Fig. 7.2

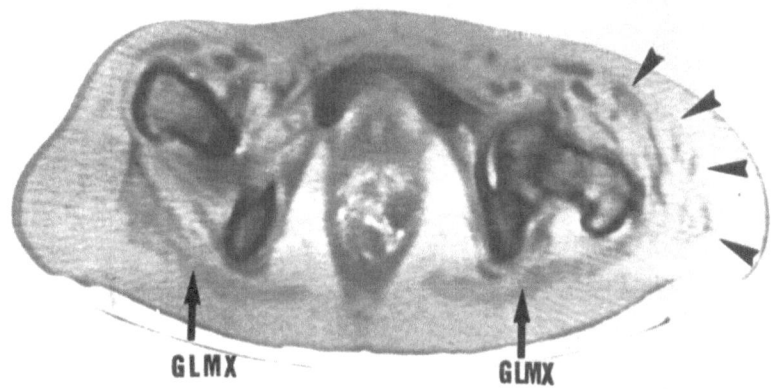

GLMX   GLMX

Fig. 7.3

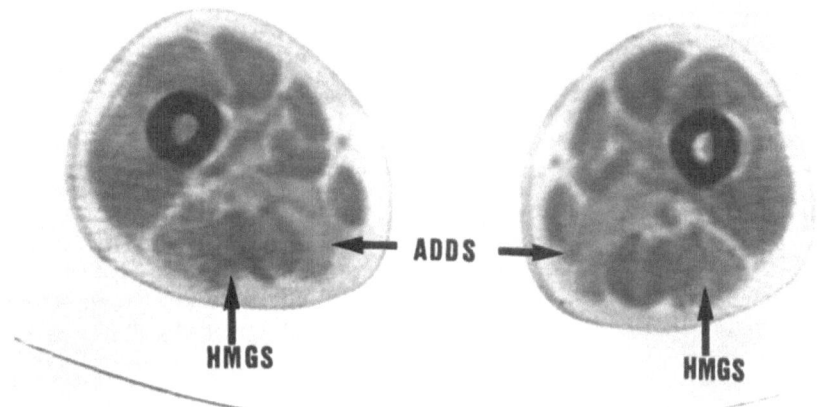

ADDS

HMGS   HMGS

Fig. 7.4

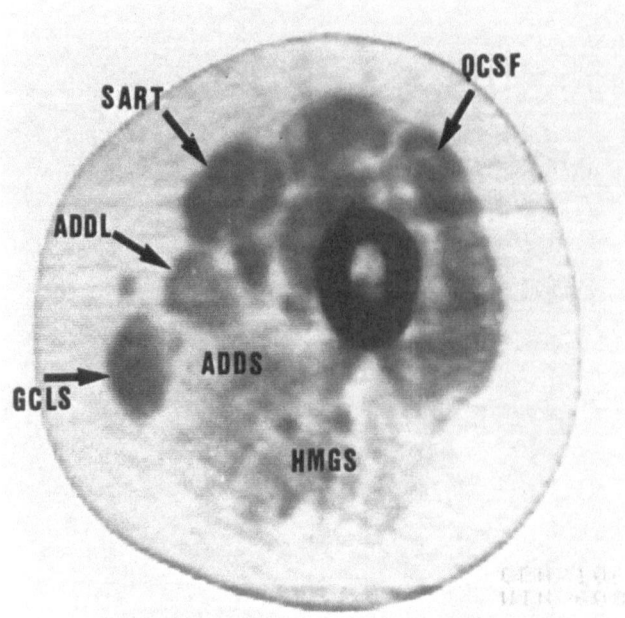

Fig. 7.5. This 18-year-old boy with typical Kugelberg-Welander spinal muscular atrophy illustrates well the ragged disintegration of the mm. adductores (*ADDS*) and hamstrings (*HMGS*). Note again the large panniculus adiposus. M. quadriceps femoris (*QCSF*), m. sartorius (*SART*), m. gracilis (*GCLS*) and m. adductor longus (*ADDL*) are still visible as separate entities

▶

Fig. 7.6. A Pelvic muscles in complete involution; 32-year-old female with chronic spinal muscular atrophy. The fascia outlines are fibrotic and deep within the panniculus adiposus. **B** The thigh muscles represent a charachteristic image: small islands of ragged muscular remnants within a "sea" of fat tissue. The patient is in a stationary phase as can be seen by comparing the figure with Fig. 6.6, of the same patient almost 3 years earlier. **C** This picture illustrates again the high degree of selectivity of muscular atrophy. Both caput mediale and laterale of m. gastrocnemius (*GACS.CM* and *GACS.CL*) are well preserved, while m. soleus (*SOLS*) has been completely destroyed. The m. extensor digitorum longus (*EDPL*) has been preserved, while the normally very resistant m. flexor digitorum longus (*FDPL*) has disappeared. M. peroneus longus (*PERL*) is severely affected. Bar = 5 cm

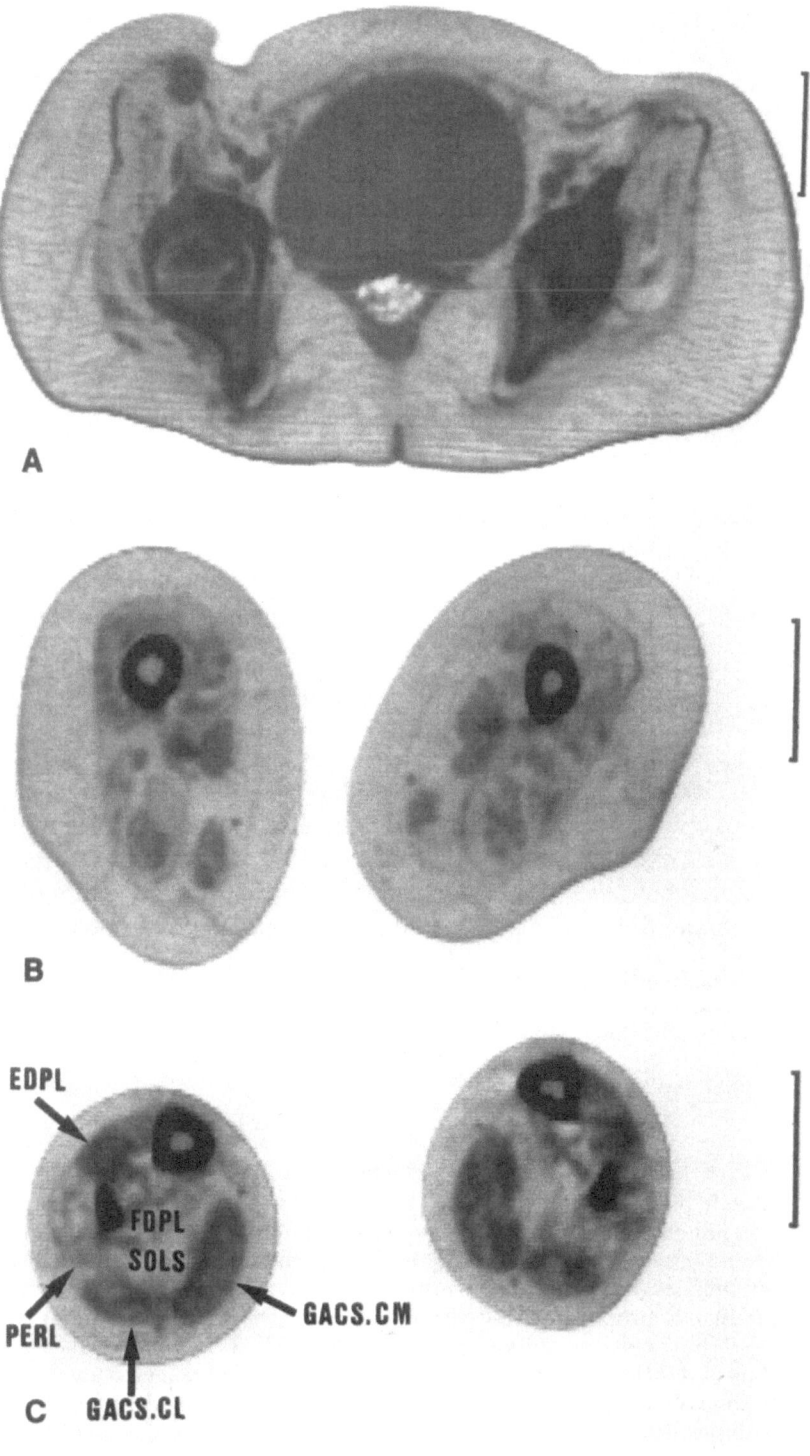

Fig. 7.6 A–C

7.2 Peripheral Radiculoneuropathies

In the classification by WALTON (1981), motor nerve roots and peripheral nerves are treated separately. In our discussion of the motor unit (Sect. 2.2) this distinction was not made, and in the present chapter we will present both radiculopathies and neuropathies. The causes of these diseases are innumerable, as can be seen in part from the classification already mentioned.

From a purely clinical point of view peripheral neuropathies can be subdivided into two categories. The first is polyneuropathies, in which a general metabolic disturbance such as diabetes mellitus causes a generalized involvement of peripheral nerves. The clinical symptomatology for all these causes is rather similar: distal ("glove and sock" distribution) sensory and/or motor symptoms such as paraesthesia, trophic disturbances, paresis of hand and foot muscles and decreased deep tendon reflexes. The pathology can be either purely axonal, as in most toxic, deficiency and paraneoplastic neuropathies where the nerve conductions will for a long time be normal, or mixed axonal and Schwann-cell (myelin) involvement characterized by a greater or lesser slowing of nerve conduction times. In both cases electromyography may reveal abnormal motor unit potentials at rest and abnormalities of the contraction pattern.

An example of a polyneuropathy is given in Fig. 7.7. As in spinal muscular atrophies, the first sign is always a diffuse infiltration of small patches of low-density tissue, particularly in distal muscles, which in the human skeletal muscular system is mainly seen in the lower extremities. The patches are, however, much coarser than in spinal muscular atrophies. Moreover, and this can be considered pathognomonic for a polyneuropathy rather than for spinal muscular atrophy, here and there larger areas of muscular defects are seen, probably corresponding to more severe nerve involvement in that particular territory.

── ▶

Fig. 7.7 A, B. Characteristic CT signs of polyneuropathy in a 57-year-old diabetic patient with polyneuropathy: diffuse infiltration of patches of low-density tissue within all muscles but with pathognomonic atrophic lesions well localized in certain muscles and nerve territories. **A** Diffusely present small patches of low-density tissue in many muscles, but particularly in m. gluteus maximus (*arrows*), very similar to spinal muscular atrophy; specific atrophy of both mm. obturatorii interni (*OBIN*), innervated by branches of plexus sacralis (L5-S2). **B** Lesions in m. vastus intermedius (*VAIM*) and m. rectus femoris (*RTFS*) on both sides, n. femoralis territory. **C** Circumscribed lesion (*arrow*) in the m. soleus (n. tibialis) of a 35-year-old male with polyneuropathy of not yet determined aetiology. Note the moth-eaten aspect of all muscles. Bar = 5 cm

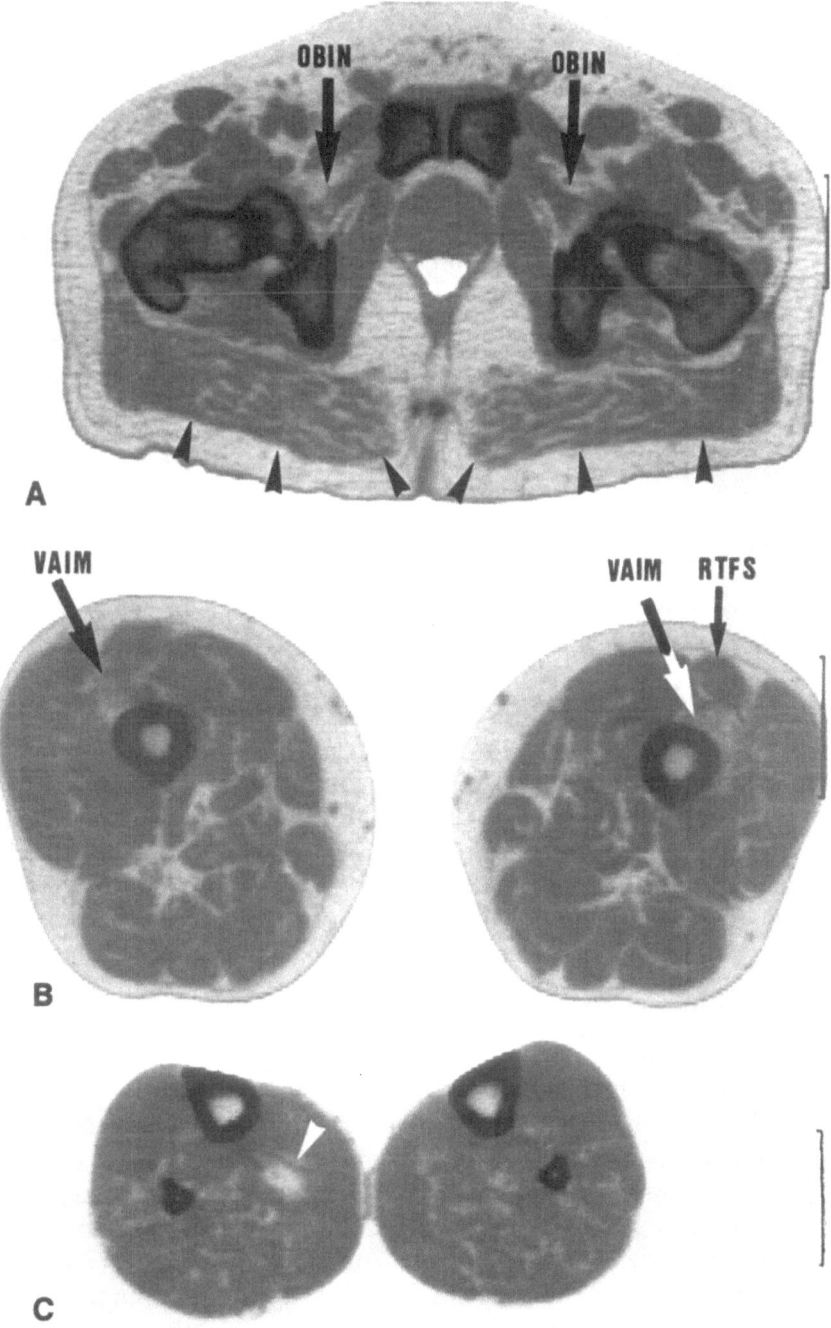

Fig. 7.7 A–C

A second category of peripheral neuropathies with or without nerve-root involvement concerns more or less isolated peripheral nerve lesions due for example to trauma or entrapment. In these situations the symptomatology is restricted to the territory innervated by one or more specific nerves. We have found that CT scanning is particularly useful and revealing in the latter category because many of these lesions are small and difficult to detect clinically or even on electromyography; the scans are in many cases the only objective proof, often with medicolegal implications, that the patient has indeed sustained a peripheral nerve lesion. These lesions are usually very well circumscribed and fit well anatomically with the known innervation patterns as described in Tables 5.1–5.12. In Figs. 7.8–7.11 a number of cases of peripheral nerve lesions are presented.

7.3 Myasthenia Gravis

Myasthenia gravis is a disease of the neuromuscular junction caused by the formation of antibodies against the acetylcholine receptor molecules on the postsynaptic membrane. These antibodies can be measured in the serum of a large number of patients (LINDSTROM et al. 1976) and immune complexes can be demonstrated at the level of the neuromuscular junctions themselves (A. G. ENGEL et al. 1977 a, b). Although this discovery and its consequences for diagnosis and therapy of myasthenia gravis constitute one of the most fascinating recent developments in the field of myopathies (A. G. ENGEL 1979), very few structural changes have been reported in the musculature of these patients, not least because myasthenia gravis is one of the few myopathies in which muscular biopsy is not a necessary examination, except perhaps for the study of the subterminal axonal ramifications as described by COËRS and DESMEDT (1959). In the almost 30 cases of myasthenia gravis in which CT scans of the muscles were performed (usually in association with the necessary CT scan of the mediastinum to exclude concomitant thymus pathology and secondary atrophy, particularly of the shoulder muscles), one morphological feature looked rather pathognomonic. It was a rather coarse, marble-like linear pattern of low-density tissue between the muscles (Fig. 6.4), which is also seen in polymyositis (Fig. 6.3). Because older reports stressed the importance of lymphocyte infiltration in muscles of patients with myasthenia gravis, in three cases contrast material was injected to see if this infiltrate could be enhanced in a specific way. One of these experiments is documented in Fig. 7.12 and must be considered negative. There are no other specific features seen on CT scans of the muscles of myasthenia gravis patients.

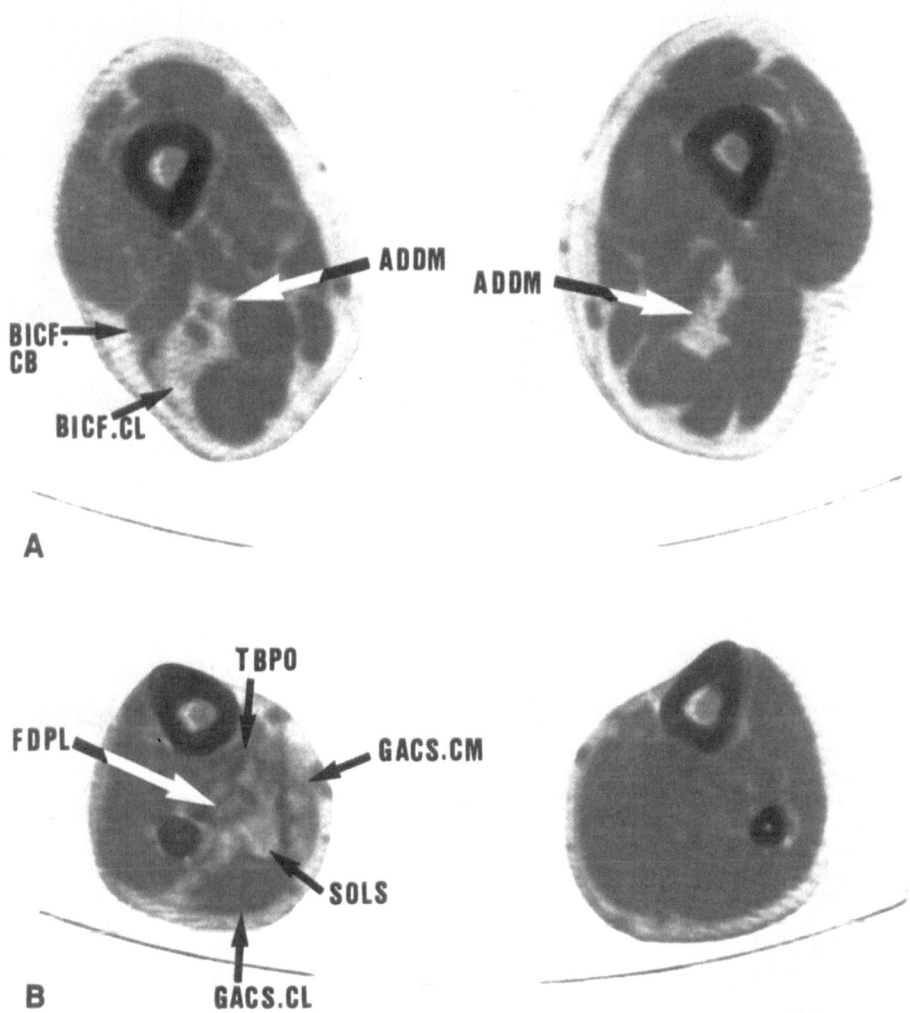

Fig. 7.8 A, B. Fifty-eight year old patient with chronic lymphadenosis; images il-lustrate mononeuritis multiplex. **A** Bilateral involvement of m. adductor magnus (*ADDM*) (n. obturatorius territory). On the right side an additional lesion of m. tibi-alis is seen, with involvement of the m. biceps femoris, caput longum (*BICF.CL*). In **B** there is involvement of m. gastrocnemius, caput mediale and laterale (*GACS.CM* and *GACS.CL*), m. soleus (*SOLS*), m. tibialis posterior (*TBPO*) and m. flexor digi-torum longus (*FDPL*). Caput breve of m. biceps femoris (*BICF.CB*) is not involved, because it is innervated by n. peroneus communis which shows no other lesions

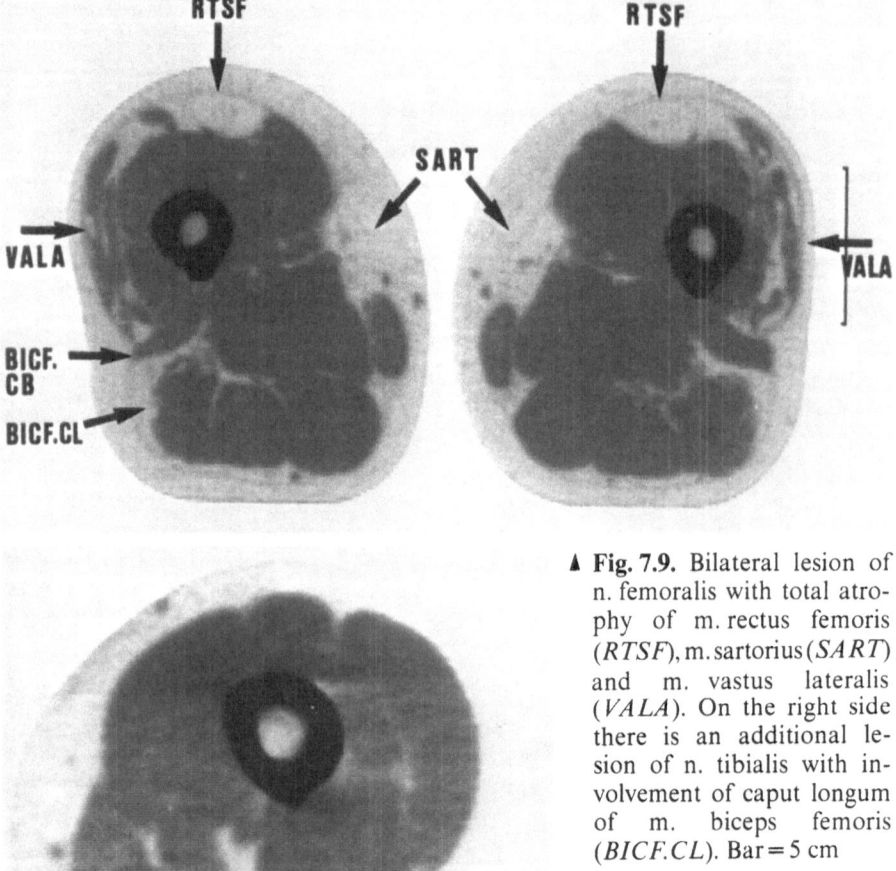

▲ **Fig. 7.9.** Bilateral lesion of n. femoralis with total atrophy of m. rectus femoris (*RTSF*), m. sartorius (*SART*) and m. vastus lateralis (*VALA*). On the right side there is an additional lesion of n. tibialis with involvement of caput longum of m. biceps femoris (*BICF.CL*). Bar = 5 cm

◀ **Fig. 7.10.** Traumatic lesion of n. tibialis affecting only the caput longum of m. biceps femoris (*BICF.CL*). The caput breve (*BICF.CB*), innervated by n. peroneus communis, is preserved and hypertrophic

Fig. 7.12 A, B. Sixty-four year old patient with myasthenia gravis. Nothing very remarkable is seen in the CT scans except the "marble-like" aspect of the lower extremities as described in Fig. 6.4. In order to check the possibility of visualizing the presumed lymphocyte infiltration in the muscles, contrast material used for brain scanning was injected and a new scan made approximately 30 min after the first. Density measurements in five locations in the m. quadriceps before contrast were 56.94 ± 5.00 HU (1 SD) on the right side and 58.64 ± 3.49 HU on the left side. After contrast the values were 61.80 ± 2.85 HU and 64.08 ± 1.48 HU. The differences are not statistically significant, but perhaps a longer impregnation period should be allowed before measuring the effect of contrast material. Bar = 5 cm

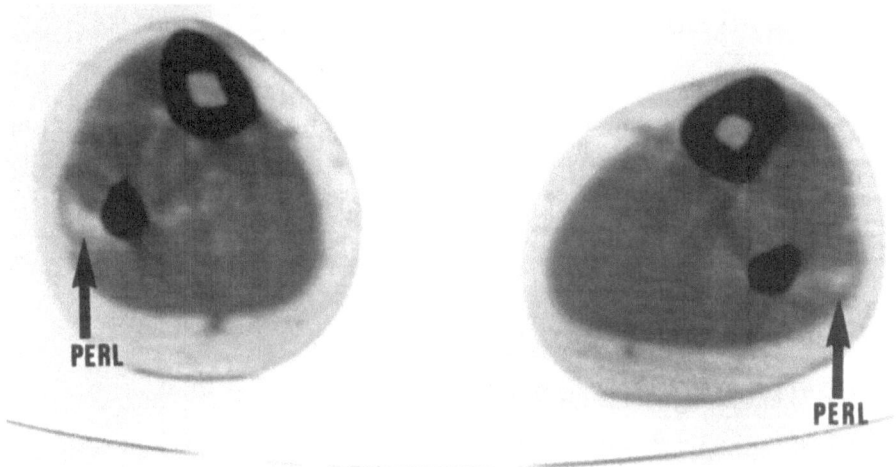

Fig. 7.11. Thirteen-year-old boy with peroneal muscular atrophy of the Charcot-Marie-Tooth type. On both the right and the left side a gap lesion is seen at the level of m. peroneus longus (*PERL*) but on the right side it is larger. Other muscles are moth-eaten and the muscles are hypotrophic compared to the left side

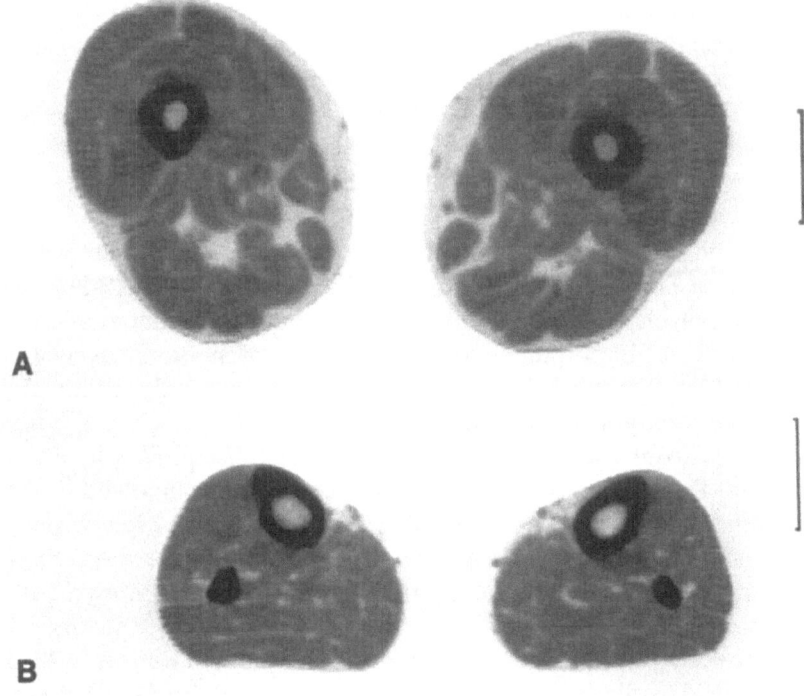

Fig. 7.12

7.4 Dystrophies

For reasons given in the introduction we will limit ourselves in this section to a more extensive description of myotonic dystrophy and of Becker's disease, together with scans of one of our longest follow-up cases, a patient with chronic polymyositis.

7.4.1 Myotonic Dystrophy

7.4.1.1 What Is Myotonic Dystrophy?

At the beginning of this century myotonic muscular dystrophy was described as a separate hereditary myotonic disease (HMD) simultaneously by STEINERT (1909) and by BATTEN and GIBB (1909). Three years later, CURSHMANN (1912) published his classical paper indicating the involvement of the endocrine system in this disease. At that time it was the third HMD known, together with myotonia congenita (THOMSEN 1876) and paramyotonia congenita (EULENBURG 1886). In the classification by the World Federation of Neurology (1968) the disease was simply called dystrophia myotonica or myotonia atrophica but "Steinert's disease" is now probably the best-known eponym. By 1968 the number of classified HMDs had increased to six, and in the classifications of BECKER (1977), BETHLEM (1977) and LIPICKY (1979) descriptions of almost twenty different types and subtypes of HMD can now be found. Nervertheless, myotonic muscular dystrophy still stands out as probably the best-studied autosomal dominant disease. A comprehensive review of our present knowledge about this disease was written by HARPER (1979).

Although the name myotonic dystrophy seems to imply merely a myopathy, it is, in fact, a rather generalized disease with various phenotypical features, of which muscular involvement is the most prominent and characteristic. The most important symptoms and signs of myotonic dystrophy are summarized in Table 7.1. It is the myopathy which usually brings the patient to the attention of the physician. A complete work-up of a case of myotonic dystrophy will, however, involve a multidisciplinary investigation not only of the myopathy but also of the other systems involved in the disease. Some patients may be found to have the complete phenotype, while others, including family members, may have only myotonia and cataract.

The most likely cause of the multi-system involvement in myotonic dystrophy is a widespread membrane defect present in many cells and organs of the body. Abnormal phosphorylation and methylation of membrane components has been claimed in erythrocyte membranes (WONG and ROSES 1979; MOORE and APPEL 1980) but the exact biochemistry of the defect remains unknown and controversial (GAFFNEY et al. 1980). One of its consequences is thought to be a disturbance of chloride (BARCHI 1975; ADRIAN and MARSHALL 1976) and calcium conductance (PLISHKER et al. 1978) through the membranes, leading in muscle cells to myotonia which is the expression of the inability of the muscle cell membrane to re-establish quickly the resting membrane potential after contraction. The sustained depolarization leads to delayed muscular relaxation, of the hand grip for example, and to the typical, prolonged contraction signal on electromyography. Myotonia can be treated with acetazolamide (KWICIENSKI 1980) and with other compounds such as baclofen (GUILLEMINAULT 1978), quinidine and procainamide. Diphenylhydantoin seems to be the drug of choice (GRIGGS et al. 1975) because of its minimal cardiac complications.

7.4.1.2 CT Scanning

In this section the pattern of muscular changes which take place during the course of myotonic dystrophy has been reconstructed by comparing 20 CT scans of 12 myotonic dystrophy patients of different ages. The youngest patient in this series had his first scan at the age of 18 years, and the oldest patient scanned was 67 years of age. All patients had a full investigation at hospital admission and they all had most of the symptoms and signs described in Table 7.1.

Although it has not been possible to verify the evolution of the muscular changes as described here in any individual patient, because our longest follow-up so far is only 42 months, we do feel that the information obtained from these cases is significant enough to give a clear impression of how this myopathy proceeds over the years.

The earliest finding in this myopathy, generally considered pathognomonic, is atrophy of the mm. sternocleidomastoidei; it may be unilateral at the onset and is usually present before atrophy becomes obvious in any other muscle. As the disease progresses, both mm. sternocleidomastoidei become increasingly hypotrophic and the space originally occupied by them is gradually filled with low-density adipose tissue. At the same time the profile of the m. levator scapulae becomes relatively prominent and dense (Fig. 7.13).

At this early stage of the disease both muscular atrophy and hypertrophy are found to coexist. The latter is particularly prominent in the abdominal wall and spinal muscles (Fig. 7.14 A) while the first signs of muscular atrophy appear in the lower leg muscles, which may explain why myotonic dystrophy is often called a distal type of myopathy (Fig. 7.14 B).

It is known that myotonia by itself can cause muscular hypertrophy, particularly in myotonic diseases in which there is little muscle destruction, such as myotonia congenita. In myotonic dystrophy muscular destruction

Table 7.1. Main symptoms and signs of myotonic dystrophy

Genetic transmission	Autosomal dominant (LYNAS 1956; KLEIN 1958) Linkage to ABO-secretor (ZIMMERLI et al. 1977)
Age at onset	15 – 35 years (neonatal) (HARPER 1975 a, b; CHASSEVENT et al. 1978; PEARCE and HÖWELER 1979)
Myopathy of cross-striated muscle	*Myotonia* always present on relaxation and/or on percussion and/or on EMG *Muscle weakness* and *atrophy* always present *Muscle hypertrophy* may be present before atrophy *Muscles clinically* involved: mm. levatores palpebrae (ptosis), m. facialis (diplegia), mm. temporales and mm. masseteres, mm. sternocleidomastoidei, mm. dorsi and distal muscles of the extremities (m. tibialis anterior). Shoulder and pelvic girdle muscles preserved until late in disease
Hart muscle involvement	Atrioventricular (His' bundle) conduction defects (JOSEPHSON et al. 1973; GRIGGS et al. 1975), sometimes leading to sudden death (MOTTA et al. 1979), are frequent
Respiratory muscle involvement	Usually minimal (GILLAIN et al. 1964; BOSSEN et al. 1974; DE BACKER et al. 1976; CARROLL et al. 1977)
Laboratory findings	Muscle enzymes usually not very indicative. Low IgG, due to hypercatabolism, frequently found (ROBERTS and BRADLEY 1977; LARSEN et al. 1980)
Smooth muscle involvement	Many symptoms of various levels of the GI tract have been described (BOSMA and BRODIE 1969; ORNDAHL et al. 1973; WEINER 1978; THÉODORE et al. 1980)
Eye lens	Cataract found in 90% of patients by slit-lamp examination (DARK et al. 1977)
CNS involvement	Mental defects and deterioration, apathy and anosognosia are very common (CAUGHEY and MYRIANTHOPOULOS 1963). EEG and brain CT scan sometimes abnormal but usually not specific ERG may be abnormal (BETTEN et al. 1971) Respiratory centre depression may cause high risk during general anaesthesia (WALD 1975)
Endocrine system involvement	Growth hormone disturbances (CULEBRAS 1977) Testicular atrophy and menstrual disturbances frequent (SAGEL et al. 1975) Hypothyroidism frequent (TREDICI and COLETTI 1978) Hyperinsulinism leading to diabetes mellitus frequent (BARBOSA et al. 1974; NUTTAL et al. 1974; KÜHN and FIEHN 1978; FESTOFF and MOORE 1979)
Peripheral nerve involvement	Frequently present (POLLOCK and DYCK 1976; PANAYITOPOULOS and SCARPALESOS 1976; OLSON 1978)
Radiological manifestations of skull	Hyperostosis, small sella with ossification of diaphragma sellae and arched palate may be found
Frontal alopecia	Very frequently present. Together with the facial diplegia and the atrophy of mm. temporales and mm. masseteres this gives many patients a haggard appearance

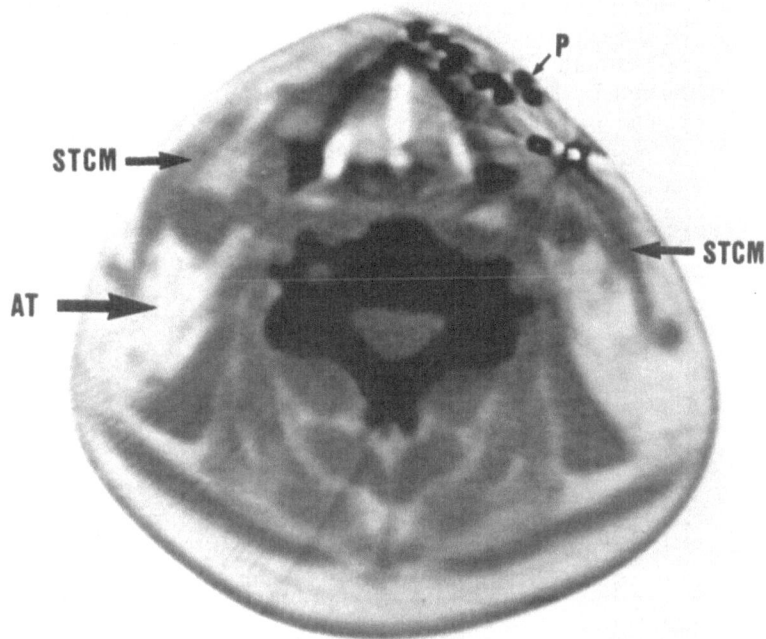

Fig. 7.13. Neck muscles of a 44-year-old male. Both mm. sternocleidomastoidei (*STCM*) are hypotrophic and the space originally occupied by them is filled up with low-density adipose tissue (*AT*). A number of shotgun pellets (*P*) are lodged between skin and platysma on the left side. On admission this patient claimed that during the war a bullet passed through his neck from the right anterior to the left posterior region where he thought he could describe the exit scar

and weakness supersede the hypertrophy and myotonia. The relative selectivity of muscular atrophy and hypertrophy found in this disease is difficult to explain. One of the first pathological findings in myotonic dystrophy is the discrepancy between the usually abnormally small type I fibres and the abnormally large types II A and II B fibres (DUBOWITZ and BROOKE 1973), but how this would selectively affect or spare certain muscles or parts of muscles, as will be described, is difficult to understand.

At this stage of the disease, in our series from the age of 30 years on, a second process sets in: atrophy of the extensor muscles of the spine (mm. dorsi), and in particular of the deeper layers of the oblique back muscles (m. transversospinalis) and of the m. extensor spinae. The atrophy seems to originate in the thoracolumbar area (Figs. 7.15, 7.16) and to spread upwards through the shoulder region to reach the cervical region later in the disease. This process of atrophy of the deep muscles of the back continues over many years, finally destroying all of the extensor muscles. The m. levator scapulae seems to be the last muscle in all cases to resist the atrophy (Figs. 7.17, 7.18).

Fig. 7.15. Abdominal and spinal muscular level in a 43-year-old male. Muscular hy- ►
pertrophy is not present and the relationship between abdominal cavity and the
muscles is here significantly different from that in Fig. 14 A. This can be due in part
to atrophy of the mm. recti abdominis (*RCAB*) which causes pseudo-obesity. At the
same time the mm. dorsi become affected, starting with the mm. interspinales
thoracis (*ISTH*) and m. multifidus (*MFDS*). Bar = 5 cm

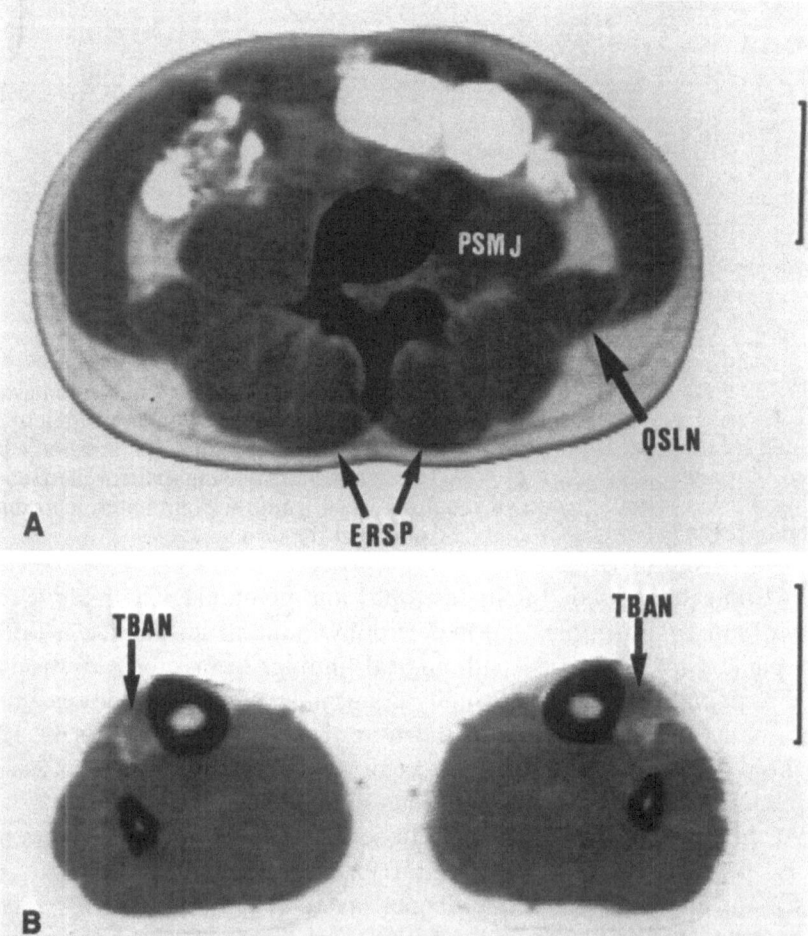

Fig. 7.14. A Abdominal and spinal muscles in a 45-year-old male. Hypertrophy of
all muscles is seen, particularly of the m. erector spinae (*ERSP*), m. quadratus lumborum (*QSLN*) and m. psoas major (*PSMJ*). These three muscles form a massive
column around the spine, and together with the hypertrophy of the abdominal wall
muscles constitute approximately three-quarters of the total surface of the abdomen.
B Lower leg muscles of the same patient, where the first signs of muscular wasting
are seen in m. tibialis anterior (*TBAN*) on both sides. Bar = 5 cm

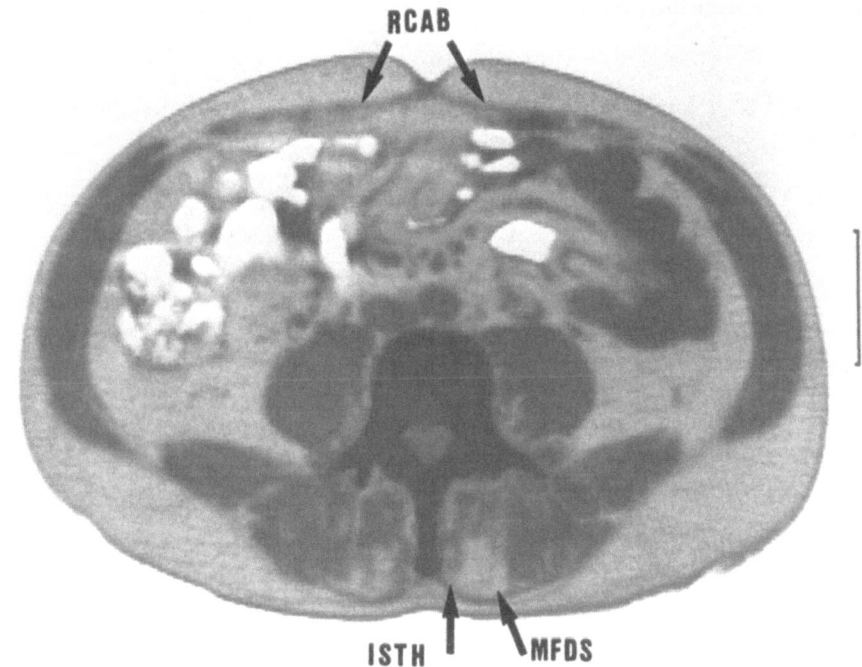

Fig. 7.15

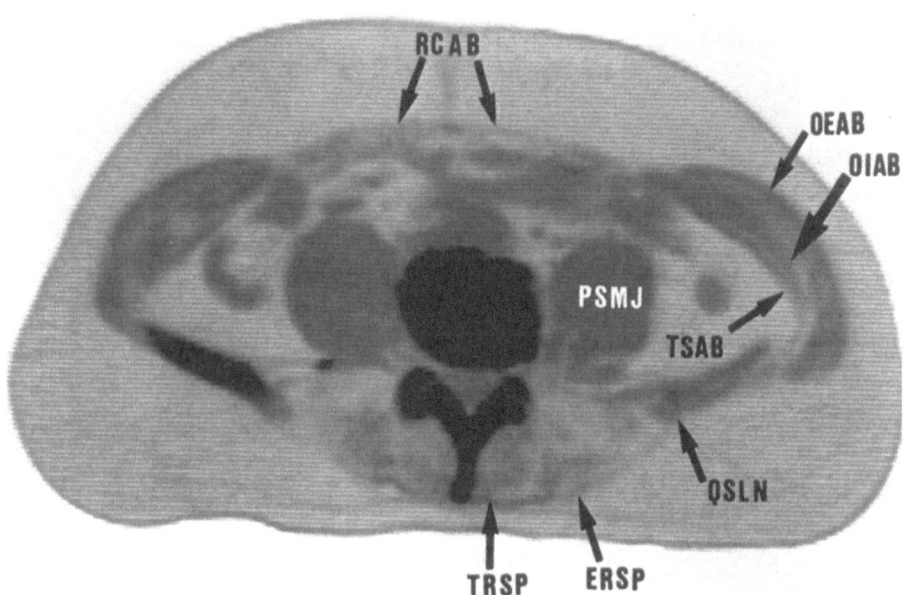

Fig. 7.16. Same level as in Fig. 7.15, in a 54-year-old male. M. transversospinalis (*TRSP*), m. erector spinae (*ERSP*) and m. quadratus lumborum (*QSLN*) are all very atrophic. The abdominal wall muscles (m. transversus abdominis (*TSAB*), m. obliquus internus abdominis (*OIAB*), m. obliquus externus abdominis (*OEAB*) and mm. recti abdominis (*RCAB*)) are infiltrated with low-density tissue, while of the large column of muscles seen in Fig. 7.14 only the m. psoas major (*PSMJ*) remains

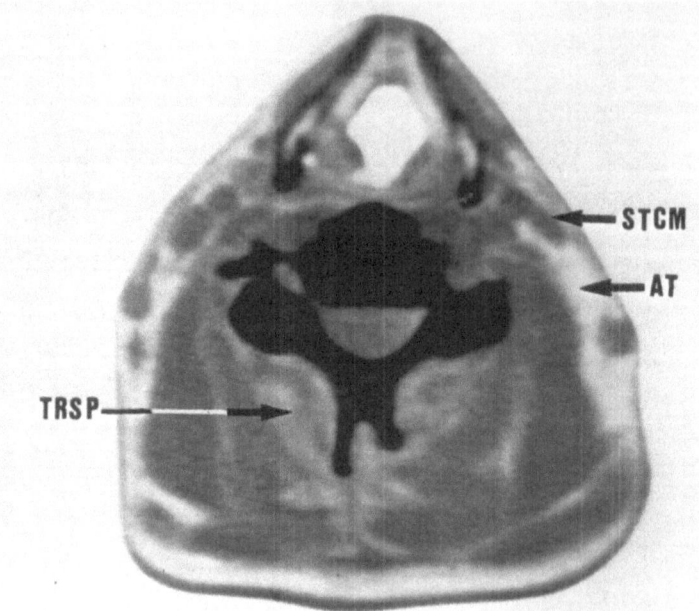

Fig. 7.17

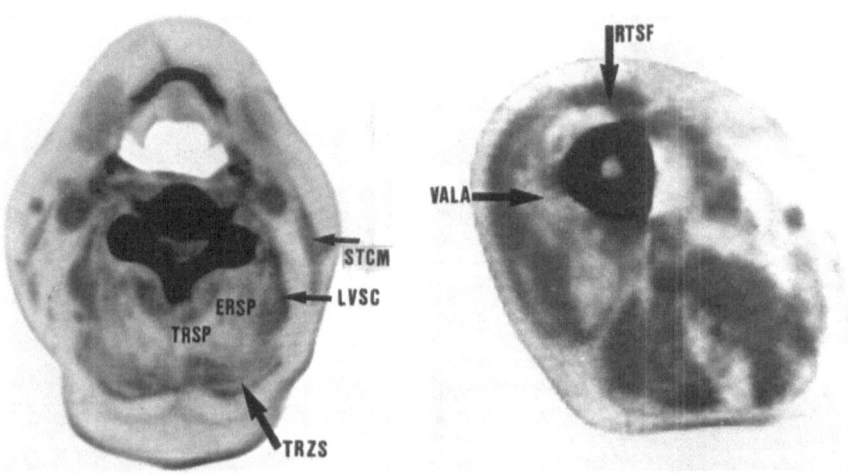

Fig. 7.18   Fig. 7.20

Fig. 7.17. Scan of the neck muscles of a 47-year-old male. Atrophy of the mm. sternocleidomastoidei (*STCM*) and adipose tissue replacement (*AT*) is almost complete. Atrophy of the m. transversospinalis (*TRSP*) is clearly evident

Fig. 7.18. Neck muscles of a 56-year-old female. Extensive destruction of the m. transversospinalis (*TRSP*) and m. erector spinae (*ERSP*) is now evident, while remnants of the mm. sternocleidomastoidei (*STCM*), m. trapezius (*TRZS*) and m. levator scapulae (*LVSC*) can still be seen

Fig. 7.20. Thigh muscles of a 53-year-old patient, enlarged to show the remarkable excavation-type atrophy of m. vastus lateralis (*VALA*). The m. rectus femoris (*RTSF*) has also become atrophic at this stage

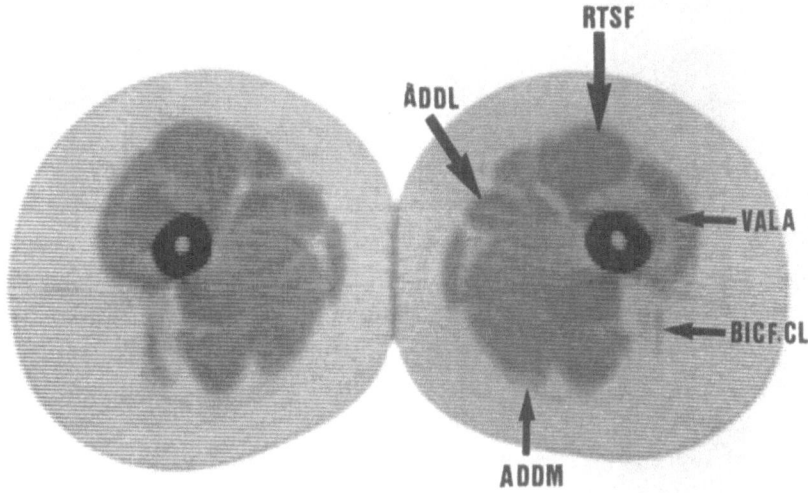

Fig. 7.19. Thigh muscles of a 34-year-old female. The onset of atrophy in m. vastus lateralis (*VALA*), predominantly on the left side, and bilateral hypertrophy of m. rectus femoris (*RTSF*) can clearly be seen. Hypertrophy of m. adductor magnus (*ADDM*) and m. adductor longus (*ADDL*) is still present. Marked atrophy of caput longum of m. biceps femoris (*BICF.CL*) is seen

While this slow process in the mm. dorsi continues, an elaborate transformation takes place in the lower extremities. We follow it here over a period of 42 months in one female patient. Figure 7.19 represents a scan of the thigh muscles done when she was 34 years of age. Hypertrophy of m. abductor magnus and longus can be observed, and very strikingly also of m. rectus femoris, most probably constituting compensatory hypertrophy for the atrophy of m. quadriceps. Atrophy of the m. quadriceps in myotonic dystrophy progresses in a very specific and peculiar pattern. The general impression is that the m. quadriceps is excavated from the inside towards the outside, starting with the m. vastus intermedius, progressing into the m. vastus lateralis and finally involving the whole muscle, leaving only an outer shell (Fig. 7.20). During most of this process, the m. rectus femoris remains relatively well preserved and is even hypertrophic in some cases.

The muscles of the lower leg become atrophic almost synchronously with the atrophic process in the m. quadriceps. The atrophy begins with the m. tibialis anterior and the caput mediale of the m. gastrocnemius, progresses to the caput laterale of the latter muscle, and finally destroys the m. soleus and all of the m. triceps surae until only the deep and most lateral muscles remain. The whole process follows the filling-up principle (Fig. 7.21).

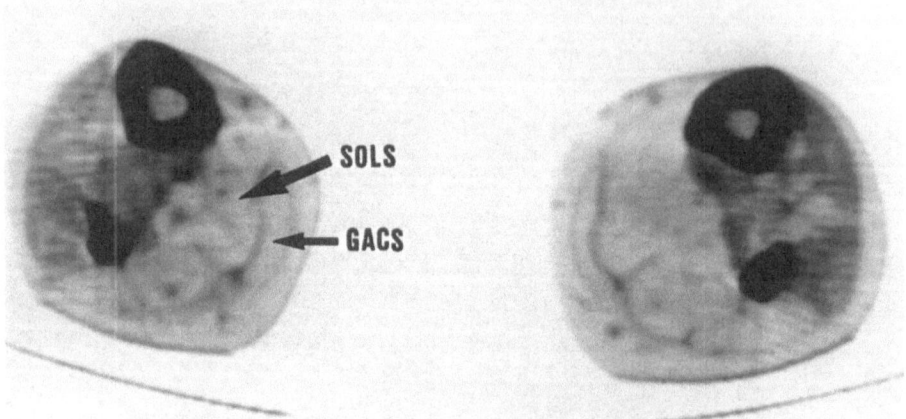

Fig. 7.21. Lower leg muscles of a 54-year-old male. Atrophy of m. gastrocnemius (*GACS*) and m. soleus (*SOLS*) has clearly followed the "filling-up" mechanism

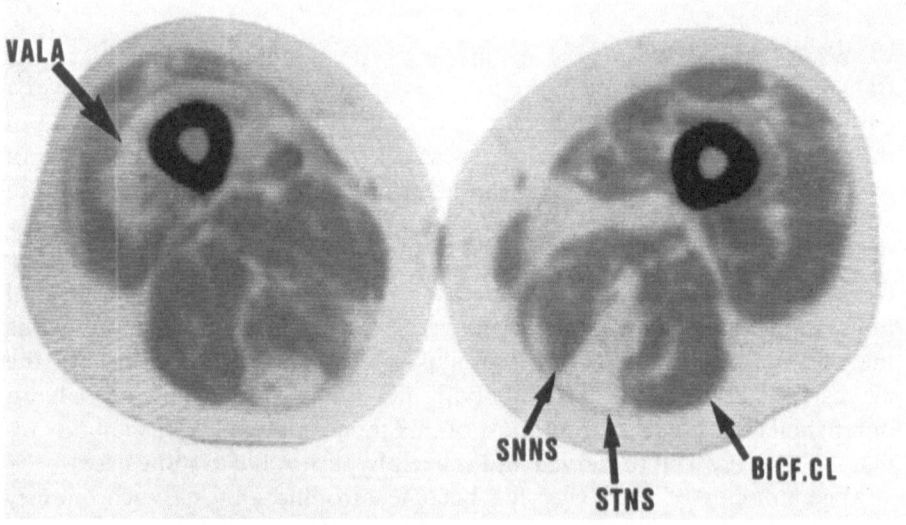

Fig. 7.22. Atrophy of the thigh muscles in a 56-year-old female The excavation of m. vastus lateralis (*VALA*) as seen in Fig. 7.20 is clearly visible, together with a pathognomonic lesion in the hamstring muscles; the fat infiltration in the m. semitendinosus (*STNS*) leaves a gap between the well-preserved m. biceps femoris (*BICF.CL*) and m. semimembranosus (*SNNS*), which is also visible in Fig. 7.20

The last muscles to become affected are the mm. adductores and the hamstrings. As seen in Fig. 7.20, a very selective sequence of events takes place, creating very typical pictures. The once hypertrophic m. adductor magnus undergoes muscular atrophy, and the mm. semimembranosus and semitendinosus have dissappeared, leaving a gap between the rest of the m. adductor magnus and the compensatory hyertrophy of the m. biceps femoris (Fig. 7.22).

The evolution which we have described can proceed very rapidly, as can be judged from Fig. 7.23, which represents the same patient as Fig. 7.19 but 42 months later. At the same time, this patient provides another example of a distal myopathy, in contrast to the proximal myopathy seen in Fig. 7.24, in a case of chronic polymyositis.

Finally, as in all neuromuscular diseases, an end-stage is reached in which all muscles are completely atrophic and only fasciae are still visible. At this stage the original diagnosis is very difficult to make on the basis of the myopathic characteristics alone.

7.4.2 Becker-Type Muscular Dystrophy

7.4.2.1 What Is Becker-Type Muscular Dystrophy?

In 1955 BECKER and KIENER reported a family with an X-linked recessive form of muscular dystrophy with later onset and slower progression than the classical X-linked muscular dystrophy of the Duchenne type (DMD). A few years later, BECKER (1962) reported two more families and reviewed 15 others from the literature. Since then the disease has been known as Becker-type muscular dystrophy (BRADLEY et al. 1978) (BMD).

Becker-type muscular dystrophy and DMD have several important features in common: transmission by the X chromosome, calf muscle (pseudo)hypertrophy and proximal pelvic muscle involvement as a first sign. BMD and DMD could therefore give the impression of being clinical variants of the same disease, as BECKER himself thought, owing to allelic genes in the same locus. Much of the literature about BMD discusses this relationship.

Since the original reports a number of clinical studies stressing the differences in symptoms and signs between the two diseases have appeared. The general consensus now is that they do represent two separate entities (BRADLEY et al. 1978; EMERY and DREIFUSS 1966; EMERY and SKINNER 1976; FILIPPI 1971; KÜHN 1979; MABRY et al. 1965; MARKAND et al. 1969; RINGEL et al. 1977; ROTTHAUWE and KOWALESKI 1966; SHAW and DREIFUSS 1969; VISSER 1981; ZELLWEGER and HANSON 1967). Some of the results of these studies, describing the main symptoms and signs of BMD, are summarized in Table 7.2.

Table 7.2. Main symptoms and signs of Becker-type muscular dystrophy

Genetic transmission	X-linked recessive Linkage to G-6PD and colour vision (EMERY et al. 1969; SKINNER et al. 1974; ZATZ et al. 1974)
Age at onset	6–18 years [mean 11.1 ± 2.8 (EMERY and SKINNER 1976)]
Myopathy of cross-striated muscle	Calf muscle hypertrophy always present early in disease. Produces pes equinus due to shortening of Achilles tendon. Gradual transition to pseudohypertrophy Muscle weakness always present and in rather standardized sequence (BECKER and KIENER 1955; BECKER 1962): m. gluteus maximus, medius and minimus first, followed by m. iliopsoas, m. quadriceps and mm. dorsi; 2–35 years after the onset also the shoulder girdle muscles involved. Distal muscles, neck muscles and muscles of the back still later. Contractures only late in disease except for Achilles tendon. Deep tendon reflexes disappear soon. Wheelchair-bound at mean age of 27.1 ± 8.4 years (EMERY and SKINNER 1976)
Heart muscle involvement	None or mild ECG abnormalities
Progression	Slow
Life expectancy	Mean age of death 42.2 ± 13.8 years (EMERY and SKINNER 1976)
Mental disturbances	Usually none or mild
Serum CK[a] range	Usually very high, especially at young age

[a] CK: creatine kinase (E.C. 2.7.3.2)

Fig. 7.23. A CT scan of the pelvic muscles of the same patient as in Fig. 7.19 but 34 months later. The three levels together represent a classical picture of distal myopathy, with atrophy most pronounced in **C**. This stands in sharp contrast to a case of proximal myopathy as shown in Fig. 7.24. **B** Atrophy with excavation of the m. quadriceps femoris (*QCSF*) is now almost complete. The septum (*S*) between the m. vastus intermedius and the other parts of the m. quadriceps femoris is clearly visible, together with the residual shell of muscle tissue of the m. vastus lateralis (*VALA*). The m. rectus femoris (*RTSF*) is remarkably well preserved. The hamstrings (*HMGS*) are relatively well preserved. **C** Only the m. flexor digitorum longus (*FDPL*), m. peroneus longus (*PERL*), and m. extensor digitorum longus (*EDPL*) are still visible. M. tibialis anterior (*TBAN*) is completely atrophic. Bar = 5 cm

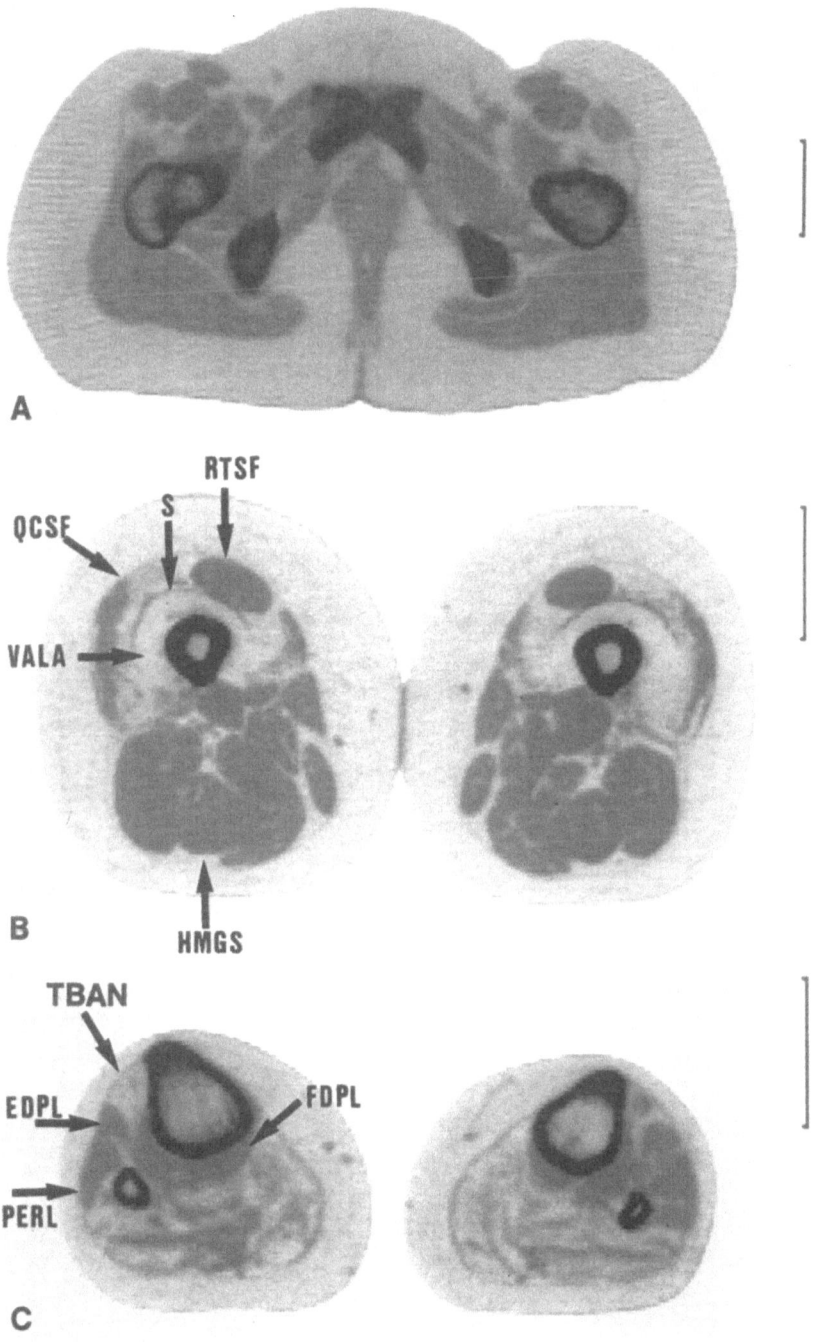

Fig. 7.23 A–C

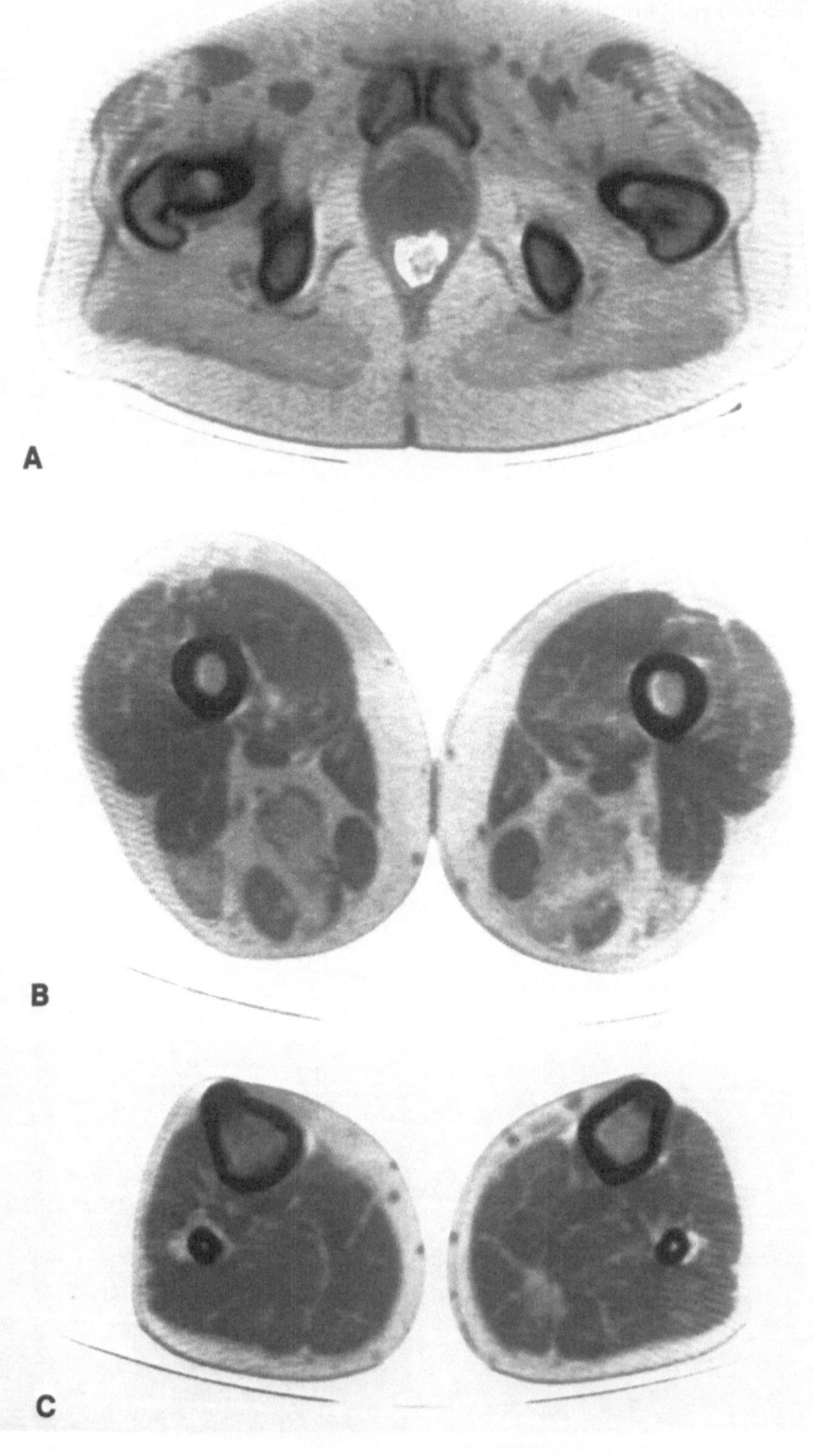

A

B

C

Table 7.3. Sequence of muscular paresis in BMD

1. m. gluteus maximus, medius and minimus
2. m. iliopsoas, m. quadriceps, mm. dorsi
3. m. tibialis anterior, mm. supra- and infraspinati
4. m. pectoralis major (pars sternocostalis), m. latissimus dorsi, m. rhomboideus, m. serratus anterior, m. trapezius (pars ascendens and transversus), m. deltoideus, mm. colli, m. biceps, m. brachioradialis, m. triceps
5. m. gastrocnemius, m. soleus
6. m. supinator, extensors of hand and fingers
7. Intrinsic hand and foot muscles, m. sternocleidomastoideus

The three main differences between BMD and DMD are summarized by EMERY and SKINNER (1976). The first is the mean age at onset, which is 11.1 ± 2.8 years for BMD and 2.8 ± 1.5 years for DMD. The second and most important is the age of becoming wheelchair-bound, which is 27.1 ± 8.4 years for BMD and 8.6 ± 1.4 for DMD. Finally, the mean age at death is 42.2 ± 13.8 years for BMD and 16.0 ± 2.7 years for DMD. These figures indicate that the progression of BMD is much slower than that of DMD.

It is now also well established that there is a separate locus on the X chromosome for each disease. Linkage studies have shown evidence that the locus for BMD is within measurable distance of the loci for colour vision and G-6PD (EMERY et al. 1969; SKINNER et al. 1974; ZATZ et al. 1974), both known to be situated on the long arm of X chromosome. Such linkage could not be demonstrated for DMD (BLYTH et al. 1965; EMERY 1966; GREIG 1977). Recent cytological studies indicate that the locus (loci?) for DMD is on the short arm of the X-chromosome (LINDENBAUM et al. 1979).

Most authors agree that BMD is less frequent than DMD, but the figures vary widely from approximately 40% (BRADLEY et al. 1978) to as low as 1% of known families with X-linked muscular dystrophy (PROT 1971); WALTON (1964) and HAUSMANOWA-PETRUSEWICZ and BORKOWSKA (1978) report 10% while MOSER et al. (1964) give an estimate of 20%.

One of the specific problems of X-linked muscular dystrophies is carrier detection. So far the best method is still the determination of creatine kinase (CK) activity in serum of carriers. At best 50%–60% of carriers can

Fig. 7.24 A–C. Typical example of a proximal myopathy, in this case polymyositis in which the proximal muscles are severely affected while the distal muscles are much better preserved. Image **C,** also shown in Fig. 6.3, can be considered rather pathognomonic for polymyositis

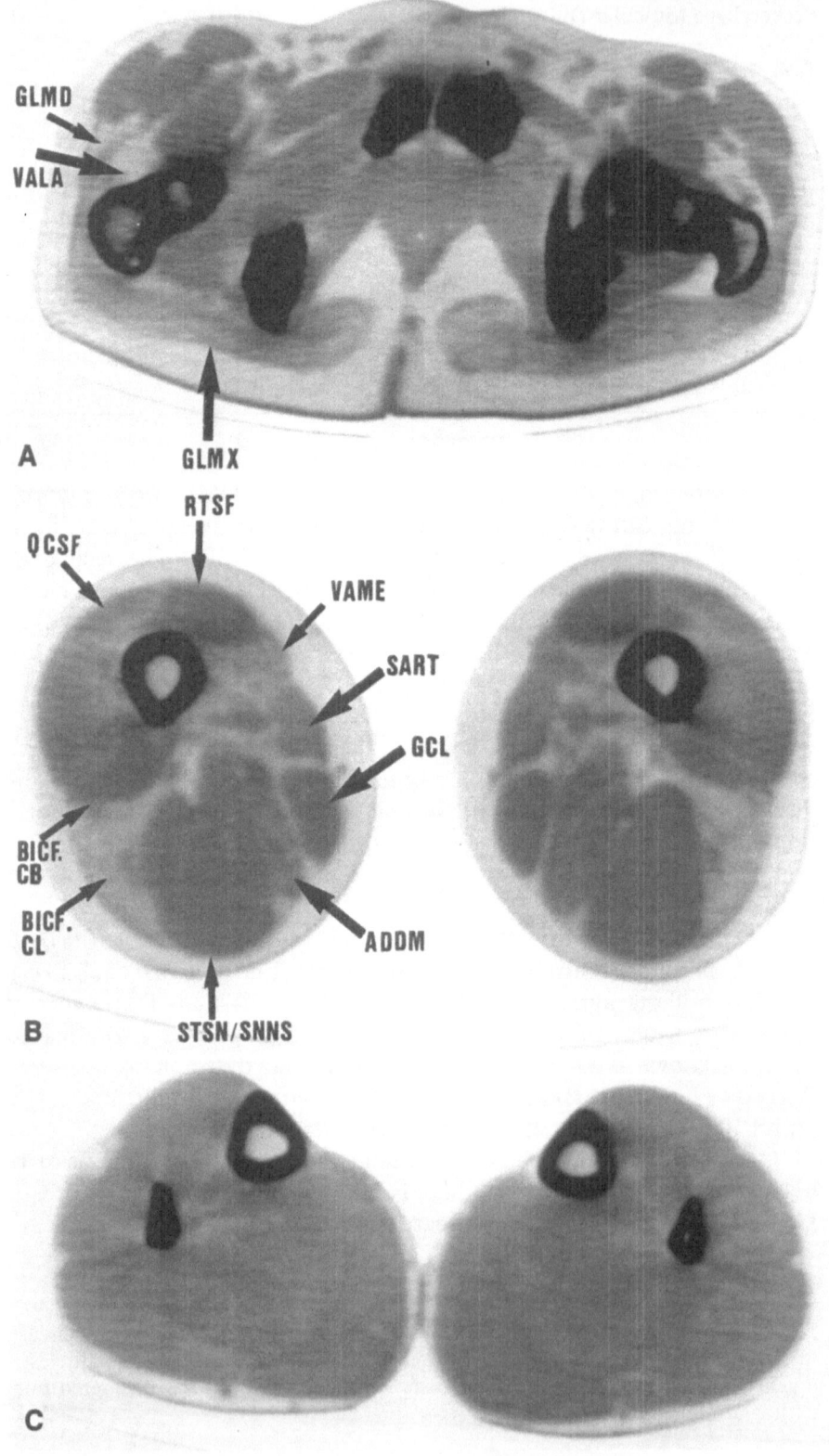

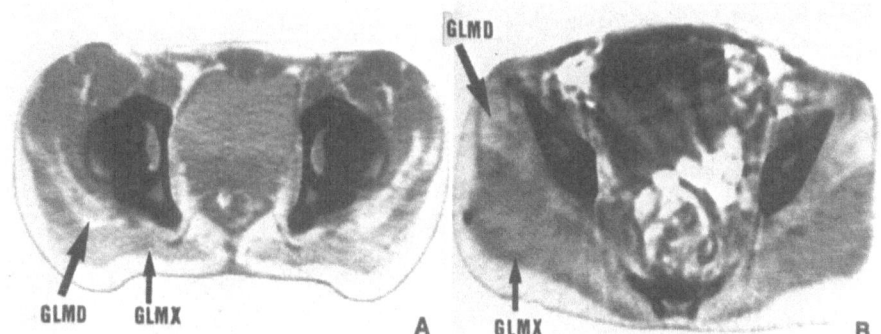

Fig. 7.26. A Nine-year-old patient with Duchenne muscular dystrophy in which m. gluteus medius (*GLMD*) is clearly more affected than m. gluteus maximus (*GLMX*). **B** The same is seen in a 10-year-old boy with the same disease. It is obvious, however, that in both m. gluteus maximus (*GLMX*) is severely involved

be detected by this method (ROTTHAUWE and KOWALESKI 1966; EMERY et al. 1967; SKINNER et al. 1975). Other methods such as examination of "lymphocyte capping" (PICKARD et al. 1979; GOLDSMITH et al. 1980) and manual testing of muscle strength (ROSES et al. 1977) are far less reliable and thus controversial (HAUSER et al. 1979).

Contractures and skeletal deformities, other than the early contracture of the Achilles tendon, occur only late in the disease (RINGEL et al. 1977; BRADLEY et al. 1978). All deep tendon reflexes disappear, beginning with the quadriceps reflexes and ending with the Achilles tendon reflexes. Several ECG abnormalities have been described, such as conduction defects, hypertrophy and dysrhythmias, but almost none in patients below the age of 20 years (MABRY et al. 1965; ZELLWEGER and HANSON 1967; MARKAND et al. 1969; WADIA et al. 1976; BRADLEY et al. 1978; HAUSMANOWA-PETRUSEWICZ and BORKOWSKA 1978). Mental disturbances were found to be either mild (EMERY and SKINNER 1976; RINGEL et al. 1977; BRADLEY et al. 1978; HAUSMANOWA-PETRUSEWICZ and BORKOWSKA 1978) or absent (ZATZ 1978).

Several authors (BECKER and KIENER 1955; BECKER 1962; EMERY and SKINNER 1976; BRADLEY et al. 1978) have described a fairly standardized sequence of muscular paresis and atrophy in BMD. BMD is perhaps the on-

---

Fig. 7.25 A–C. Twenty-four year old patient. **A** Atrophy of m. gluteus maximus (*GLMX*), m. gluteus medius (*GLMD*) and m. vastus lateralis (*VALA*) is seen. **B** Atrophy of m. quadriceps femoris (*QCSF*), and in particular m. vastus medialis (*VAME*) and m. biceps femoris, while other muscles are well preserved and even hypertrophic: m. rectus femoris (*RTSF*), m. sartorius (*SART*), m. gracilis (*GCLS*) and the m. semimembranosus (*SNNS*) and m. semitendinosus (*STNS*). The m. adductor magnus (*ADDM*) is still well preserved

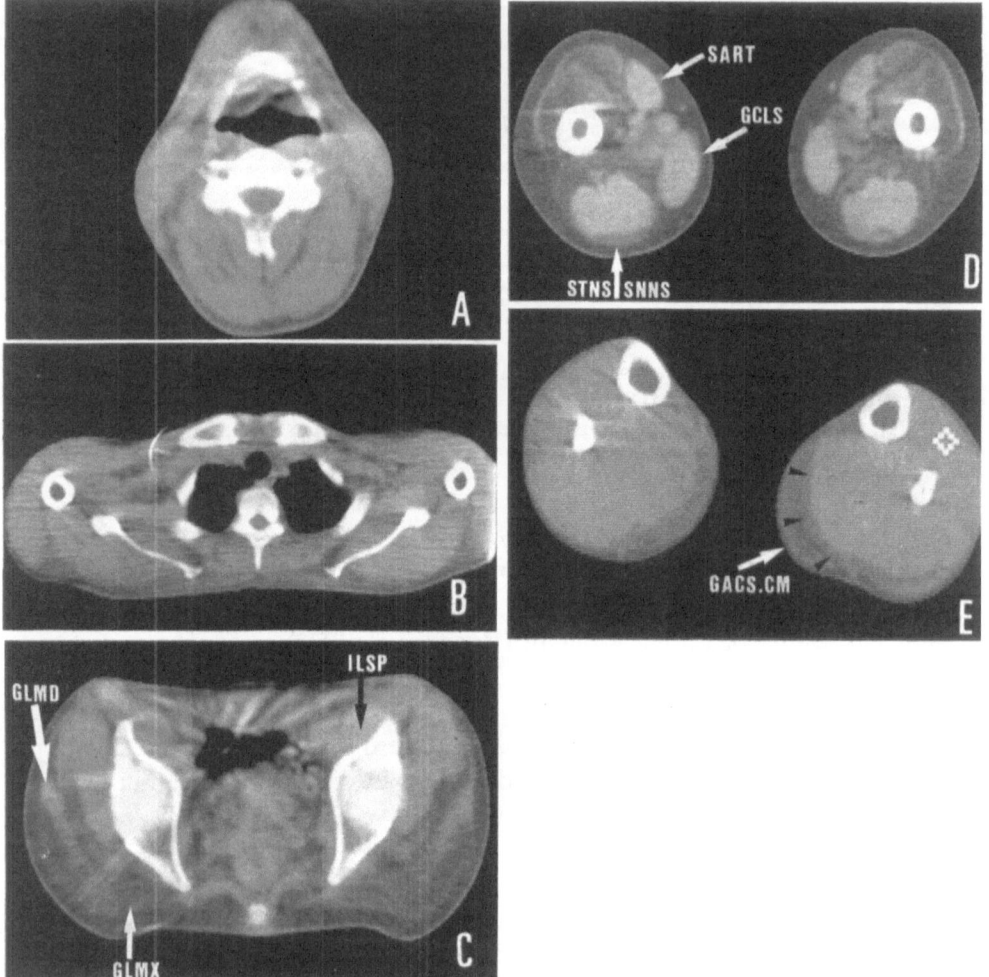

Fig. 7.27 A–E. Twenty-three year old patient with DMD shown in five levels. **A** The neck muscles and **B** the shoulder muscles are normal. In **C** the classical atrophy of m. gluteus maximus (*GLMX*) and m. gluteus medius (*GLMD*) is seen. M. iliopsoas is well preserved (*ILPS*). **D** Atrophy of all muscles with compensatory hypertrophy of m. sartorius (*SART*), m. gracilis (*GCLS*) and m. semimembranosus (*SNNS*) and m. semitendinosus (*STNS*). **E** Calf muscle hypertrophy with onset of filling-up process in m. gastrocnemius, caput mediale (*GACS.CM*)

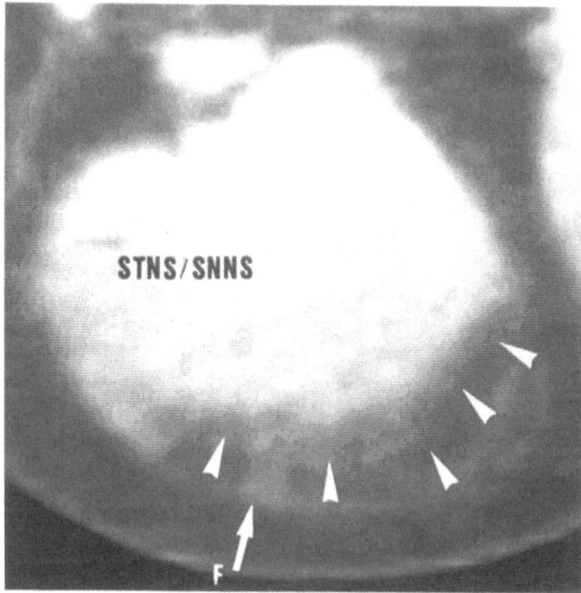

Fig. 7.28. Enlargement of the hypertrophic m. semitendinosus (*STNS*) and m. semimembranosus (*SNNS*) complex from Fig. 7.27. Low-density tissue (*arrows*) is seen to fill up inside the intact muscular fascia (*F*), causing a rather sharply delineated gap lesion

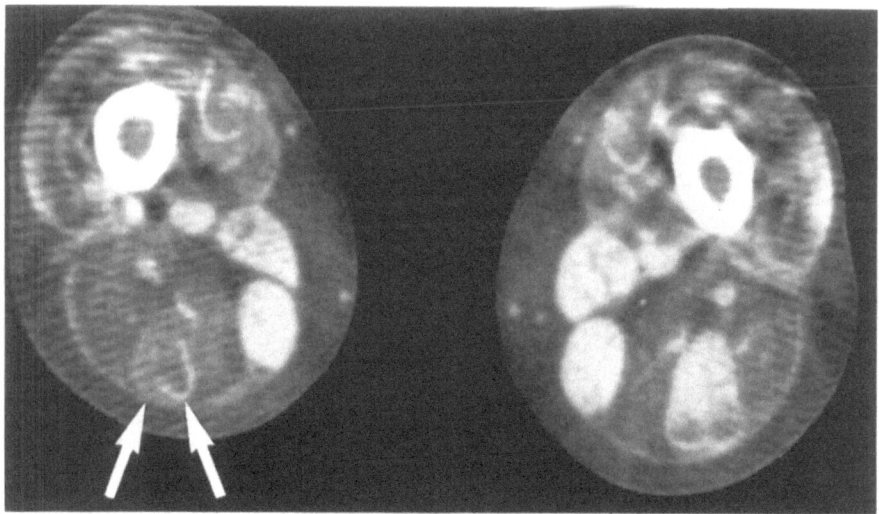

Fig. 7.29. Almost 2 years later all hamstrings have disappeared but the fascia outline (*arrows*) of the hypertrophic muscles of Fig. 7.27 is still visible

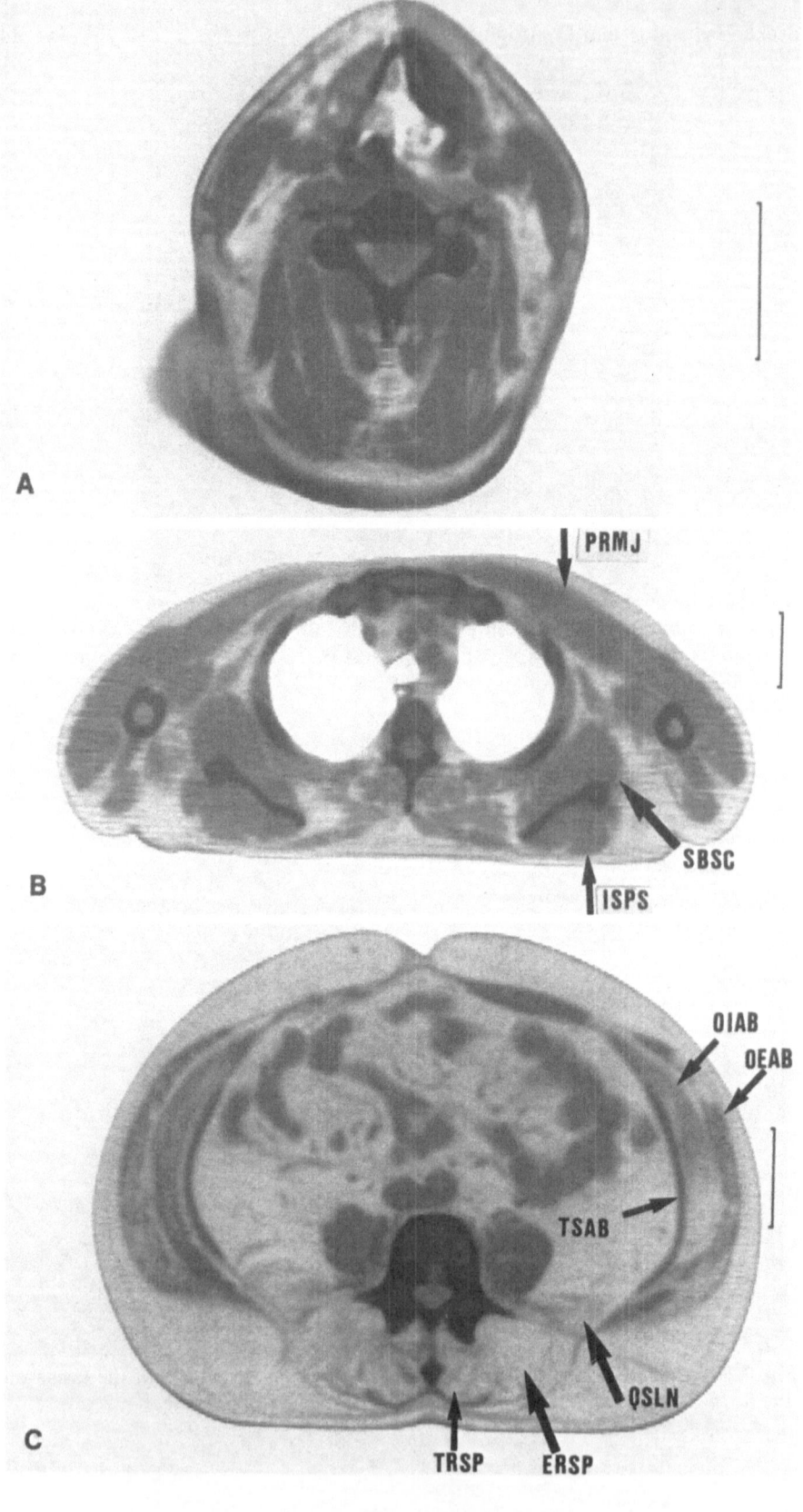

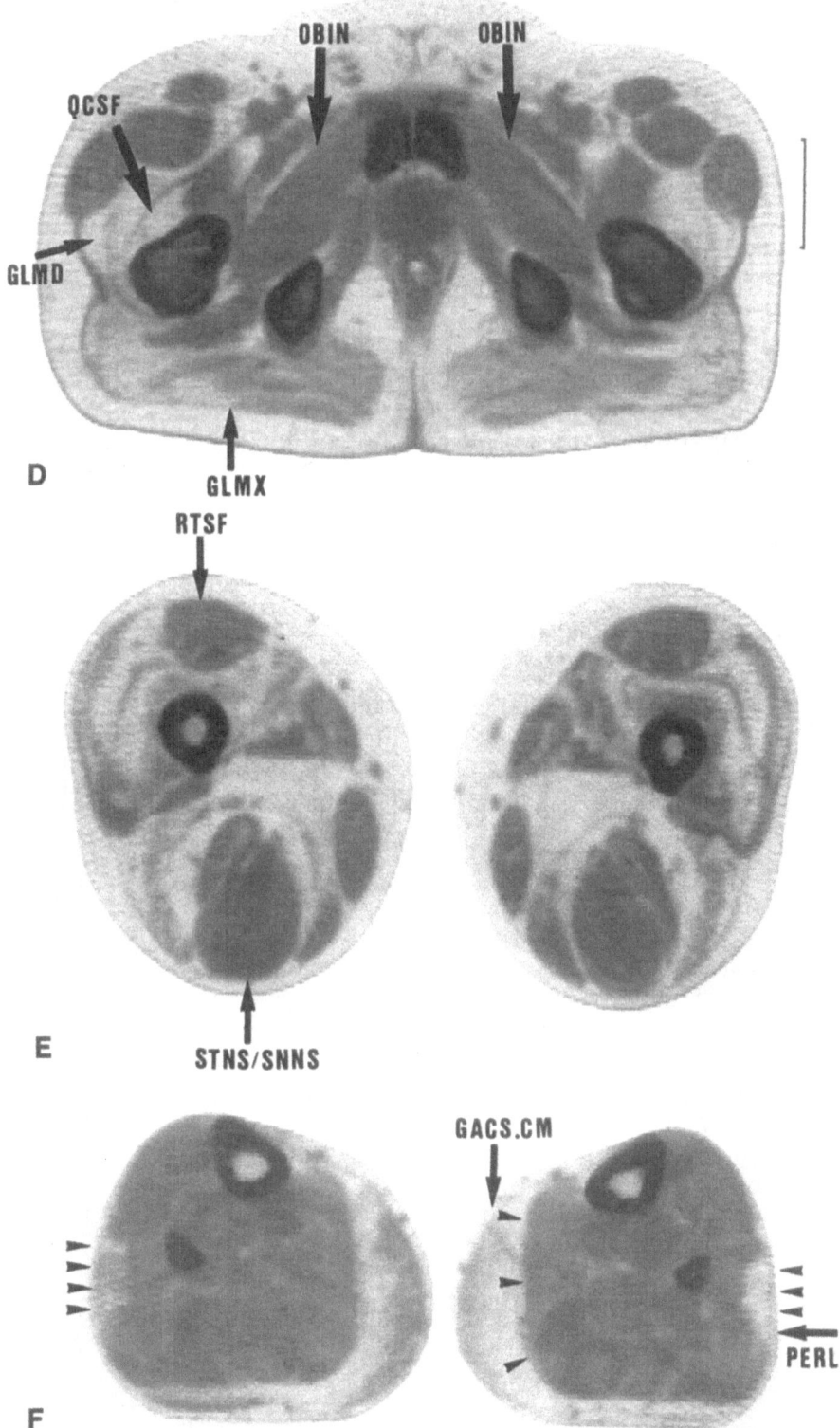

Fig. 7.30 A–F. Legend see page 146

ly myopathy for which this has been done so extensively. We have tried to reconstruct this sequence in Table 7.3 so that it can be compared in detail with the CT scan findings. All authors agree that muscular paresis starts in the pelvic girdle muscles and only later involves the shoulder muscles. In younger patients the extensor muscles seem to be affected first and flexors only later on (EMERY and SKINNER 1976). Paresis remains symmetrical in most cases. Muscular hypertrophy has been described clinically not only in the calf muscles but also in m. tensor fasciae latae, mm. dorsi, m. in-fraspinatus, m. deltoideus (BECKER and KIENER 1955; BECKER 1962), m. tri-ceps, m. biceps, m. quadriceps (BRADLEY et al. 1978), m. brachioradialis and m. gluteus maximus (DESAI et al. 1972). The muscular strength of the calf muscles remains strong until very late in the disease when pseudo-hypertrophy replaces true hypertrophy.

In the study of BRADLEY et al. (1978) a number of clinical criteria con-sidered essential for the diagnosis are summarized: (1) X-linked recessive inheritance, (2) ambulation maintained until at least 16 years of age, (3) calf pseudohypertrophy always present, (4) early contracture of the Achilles tendons and later of other muscles, (5) a specific distribution of muscle wasting of hip joint, m. tibialis anterior, mm. supra- and infraspinati, m. serratus anterior, m. pectoralis, and mm. biceps and brachioradialis, other muscles being relatively spared until later in the disease. The cases presented in this section do essentially conform with the above criteria, although we do not completely agree with the stated sequence of paresis.

Fig. 7.30A–F see pages 144 and 145

Fig. 7.30A–F. Complete picture of BMD in a 44-year-old patient. **A** Neck muscles almost normal. **B** Hypertrophy of m. pectoralis major (*PRMJ*), m. subscapularis (*SBSC*) and m. infraspinatus (*ISPS*). **C** Severe atrophy of m. transversospinalis (*TRSP*), m. erector spinae (*ERSP*) and m. quadratus lumborum (*QSLN*), atrophy of m. transversus abdominis (*TSAB*), m. obliquus internus abdominis (*OIAB*) and m. obliquus externus abdominis (*OEAB*). **D** Atrophy of m. gluteus maximus (*GLMX*), m. gluteus medius (*GLMD*) and m. quadriceps femoris (*QCFS*). Hy-pertrophy of m. obturatorius internus (*OBIN*). **E** Hypertrophy of m. rectus femoris as main extensor and m. semimembranosus (*SNNS*), m. semitendinosus (*STNS*) as main flexor. **F** Hypertrophy of lower legs but with filling-up of caput mediale of m. gastrocnemius (*GACS.CM*) and gap lesion at the level of the m. peroneus longus (*PERL*). Bar = 5 cm

Fig. 7.31A–C. Late-stage BMD in a 50-year-old patient. **A** Atrophy of most pelvic ▶ muscles except m. sartorius (*SART*) and m. iliopsoas (*ILPS*). **B** Atrophy of all muscles except m. sartorius (*SART*), m. gracilis (*GCLS*) and m. biceps femoris, caput breve (*BICF.CB*). **C** True pseudohypertrophy with low-density tissue in-filtration in enlarged m. soleus (*SOLS*); well-preserved m. tibialis posterior (*TBPO*) and m. flexor digitorum longus (*FDPL*); gap lesion of m. peroneus longus (*PERL*) and hypertrophy of m. tibialis anterior (*TBAN*)

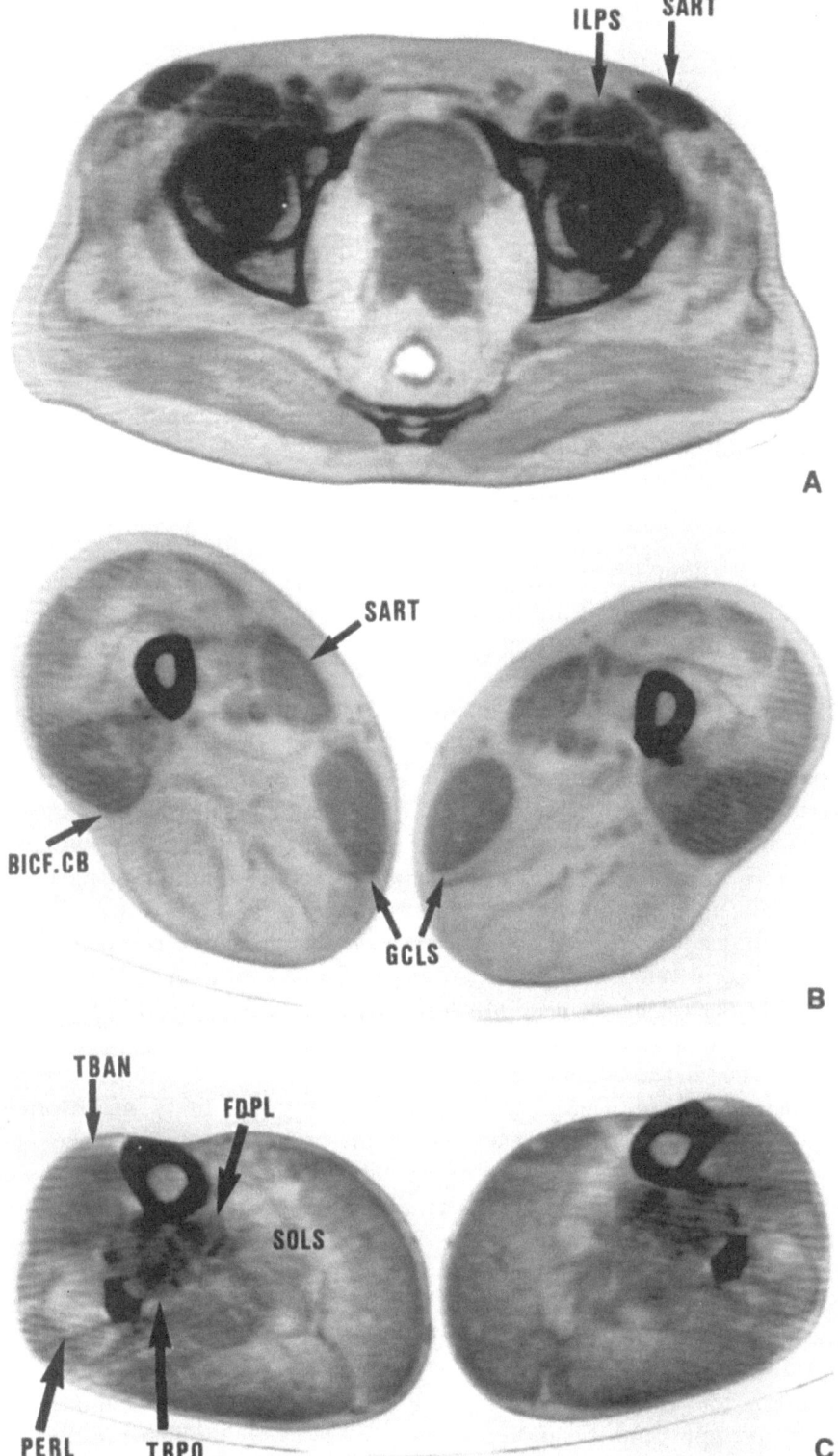

7.4.2.2 CT Scanning

A selection of pictures will be presented from 28 CT scans made in ten patients with Becker's disease. The youngest patient was first scanned at the age of 23 and the oldest at 53 years.

We will try to reconstruct from a number of CT scans obtained at different ages how muscular wasting proceeds in BMD. We have been able to verify some of these changes in individual patients on whom follow-up scans over several years could be obtained. The longest follow-up was 55 months. We also want to remind the reader that the first patient we ever scanned (Fig. 1.1) probably had the same diagnosis. It will be seen that the cases presented here are much like his. Unfortunately we have not been able to examine this first patient since.

The CT scans of BMD represent perhaps the most pathognomonic morphological picture of all the diseases we had the opportunity to examine. This is why we have opted for the presentation of only four cases, two of them with complete CT scan pictures on all levels. We have done this also because some of our atrophy findings do not correspond with the clinical analytical muscular power tests which are summarized in Table 7.3.

The first patient (Fig. 7.25) already exhibits the main chracteristics of the disease: hypertrophy of the calf muscles, a mixed pattern of atrophy and hypertrophy in the thigh muscles with a standard set of compensatory hypertrophic muscles and atrophy of m. gluteus maximus. The m. gluteus maximus is the first to show atrophy and, for the small number of cases which we have seen, this seems to be different from Duchenne muscular dystrophy where deeper layers of m. gluteus medius and minimus are systematically affected before the m. gluteus maximus (Fig. 7.26 A, B).

The transition between compensatory hypertrophy and complete atrophy is demonstrated in Figs. 7.27–7.29. In Fig. 7.27 a patient is shown in whom the disease has evolved much further than in the patient in Fig. 7.25. The neck and shoulder muscles are intact but the m. quadriceps femoris including the m. rectus femoris is severely atrophic. The mm. adductores are also atrophied. Compensatory hypertrophy is seen in m. sartorius, m. gracilis and the m. semimembranosus–m. semitendinosus complex. The lower leg muscles are still hypertrophic but invasion by low-density tissue has started at the caput mediale of m. gastrocnemius. M. gluteus medius is now also severely hypodense. In Fig. 7.28 an enlargement is shown of the m. semitendinosus–m. semimembranosus complex of the right leg. Low-density tissue infiltration has started, probably proceeding by a filling-up process, so that almost 2 years later the compensatory hypertrophy has disappeared (Fig. 7.29).

In Fig. 7.30 at 44-year-old patient is shown on all levels to demonstrate that hypertrophy and pseudohypertrophy are not only problems of the calf muscles. Hypertrophy is found on all levels and in different muscles, most of them difficult to examine clinically. This patient indeed has calf muscle hypertrophy, but also hypertrophy of m. pectoralis major, m. subscapularis, m. infraspinatus, m. obturatorius internus and m. rectus femoris. Hypertrophy is a generalized phenomenon. The second reason for presenting this case completely is to draw attention to one other intriguing finding: atrophy of m. peroneus longus, sometimes very sharply delineated, which has been found frequently and early in most cases of BMD. We have never seen atrophy of m. tibialis anterior, but have often seen this peroneus lesion with hypertrophy, essentially of m. soleus. A second case demonstrating this feature is illustrated by Fig. 7.31.

8 Correlations Between Radiological, Pathological, Muscular Power and EMG Data

8.1 Correlations Between Radiological and Pathological Data

In order to correlate radiological data, in particular the significance of density measurements, to parameters which are used in pathology to measure muscular atrophy and hypertrophy, 21 muscle biopsies taken from patients with various neuromuscular diseases (Table 8.1) were examined. The biopsies had been taken from the m. vastus lateralis exactly 15 cm above the upper edge of the patella, the level at which the CT scans are also carried out.

Density measurements were taken in the m. quadriceps, three in the m. vastus lateralis and two in the m. rectus femoris, on CT scans taken prior to the muscle biopsy. They were recorded on both the right and the left side. Because we found no significant difference between the readings in the four groups, they were pooled to ten readings per subject and the mean and standard deviation were calculated from these data. One of the problems we faced was the narrow range of the density measurements which we obtained. This was, in fact, a consequence of our method of selecting biopsy sites on CT scans, which is to take a muscle that we know to be involved but that does not have any significant fat infiltration which could be causing secondary artefacts.

The neuropathological examination of the biopsies was carried out by means of a Leitz (E. Leitz Wetzlar GmbH) ASM-Image Analysis System, which permits direct real measurements and on-line statistical analysis of cell parameters, e.g. circumference and surface area of cells and other structures such as muscular fasciculi.

Muscle biopsy sections that had been stained for ATPase at pH 9.4 were examined; this made the two main types of muscle fibres clearly visible. In a first step, a correlation was sought between the size of muscular fasciculi and density measurements. In seven cases all muscular fasciculi visible in the biopsy were measured, followed by a calculation of the mean surface area of the fasciculi. In each of the fourteen other cases only one fasciculus was studied after random selection. The relationship between density measurements and size of the fasciculi is represented in Fig. 8.1. In a second

Table 8.1. Data on patients from whom muscular biopsies were taken

Biopsy no.[a]	Initials	Sex	Age	Diagnosis
1	C. J.	M	39	Becker's disease
2	H. D.	M	11	Duchenne m.d.
3	B. H.	M	24	Becker's disease
4	C. L.	M	39	Polymyositis
5	S. N.	F	27	McArdle's disease
6	P. E.	F	23	Myopathy of aetiology n.y.d.
7	VL. L	M	44	Becker's disease
8	H. F.	F	52	Myasthenia gravis
9	D. G.	F	29	Myopathy of aetiology n.y.d.
10	G. R.	F	24	A.r. limb-girdle m.d.
11	D. N.	F	23	Myopathy of aetiology n.y.d.
12	VD. G.	F	42	Autosomal recessive s.m.a. (Kugelberg-Welander)
13	D. M.	F	25	Acute alcoholic rhabdomyolysis
14	P. M.	F	47	Myopathy of aetiology n.y.d.
15	DB. S.	F	27	Myopathy and hypothyroidism
16	M. F.	M	53	A.r. limb-girdle m.d.
17	A. J.	M	57	Quadriceps myopathy
18	F. D.	M	20	Becker's disease
19	C. B.	M	17	Myopathy of aetiology n.y.d.
20	L. L.	M	57	Myasthenia gravis
21	N. L.	M	26	Myopathy with mitochondrial abnormalities

m.d., muscular dystrophy; a.r., autosomal recessive; n.y.d., not yet determined
[a] The same numbers are used in all following figures and tables

step, measurements were made of the size of all type I and type II cells of one complete fasciculus chosen at random. The mean and standard deviation of the mean of these cases are represented in Figs. 8.2 and 8.3. Finally, in Table 8.2 correlations are represented between density measurements and atrophy and hypertrophy factors, as described by DUBOWITZ and BROOKE (1973) for type I and type II cells. In the normal m. vastus lateralis in males the muscle cells should have a diameter of between 40 and 80 μm, and in females, of between 30 and 70 μm. The atrophy factor of type I cells (A1) is obtained by making histogram of type I cells in classes of 10 μm. The classes between 40 and 80 μm are the normal cells. Those in the class 30–39 μm are given one point, those in the class 20–29 μm 2 points, and so on. One point is added per 10 μm step. The number of cells in each class is counted and multiplied by its point value. All "atrophy points" are then added together, divided by the total number of cells in the histogram

Table 8.2. Relationship between density measurements and atrophy and hypertrophy factors in m. vastus lateralis biopsies

Case no.	Density measurements (HU)	A1[a]	H1[b]	A2[c]	H2[d]
1	14.10 ± 16.24	114	2378	86	1371
2	21.30 ± 18.27	0	2000	0	1750
3	28.30 ± 19.65	0	2642	95	2503
4	30.10 ± 26.81	150	225	409	258
5	32.50 ± 13.10	0	2425	0	4321
6	38.10 ± 14.98	45	2398	0	2608
7	40.18 ± 21.16	52	922	36	2291
8	41.00 ± 8.69	0	1091	0	2459
9	41.60 ± 24.80	0	1315	3	485
10	44.90 ± 10.25	0	1900	0	1000
11	45.70 ± 8.20	41	1401	0	4120
12	46.60 ± 27.93	0	1127	0	200
13	47.01 ± 7.82	0	2	117	0
14	49.90 ± 4.40	0	2000	0	3296
15	50.20 ± 10.19	0	809	0	1403
16	50.50 ± 16.25	0	2891	0	2264
17	53.93 ± 8.98	120	0	30	60
18	54.17 ± 8.98	136	952	90	940
19	56.74 ± 5.13	0	1245	0	2046
20	57.51 ± 9.83	33	327	76	580
21	59.35 ± 4.65	20	12	18	421

[a] Atrophy factor of type I cells
[b] Hypertrophy factor of type I cells
[c] Atrophy factor of type II cells
[d] Hypertrophy factor of type II cells

and multiplied by 1000 to obtain the atrophy factor. The same applies equally to cells greater than 80 μm is diameter on which hypertrophy factors are calculated.

It is quite obvious from these results that there is no linear correlation between the density measurements, the size of fasciculi, the size of the cells and trophy and hypertrophy factors. The conclusion of these investigations has to be that a density measurement is a measure on its own, which is related to the muscle as a whole including muscle cells and non-muscular elements. It is probably determined by the amount of perimysial infiltration between the fasciculi, and says little or nothing about the pathology of the muscle cells alone. The importance of this perimysial parameter, which is not usually commented upon in routine histochemistry and certainly not in electron microscopy, was stressed by FRANTZELL and INGELMARK as early as 1951.

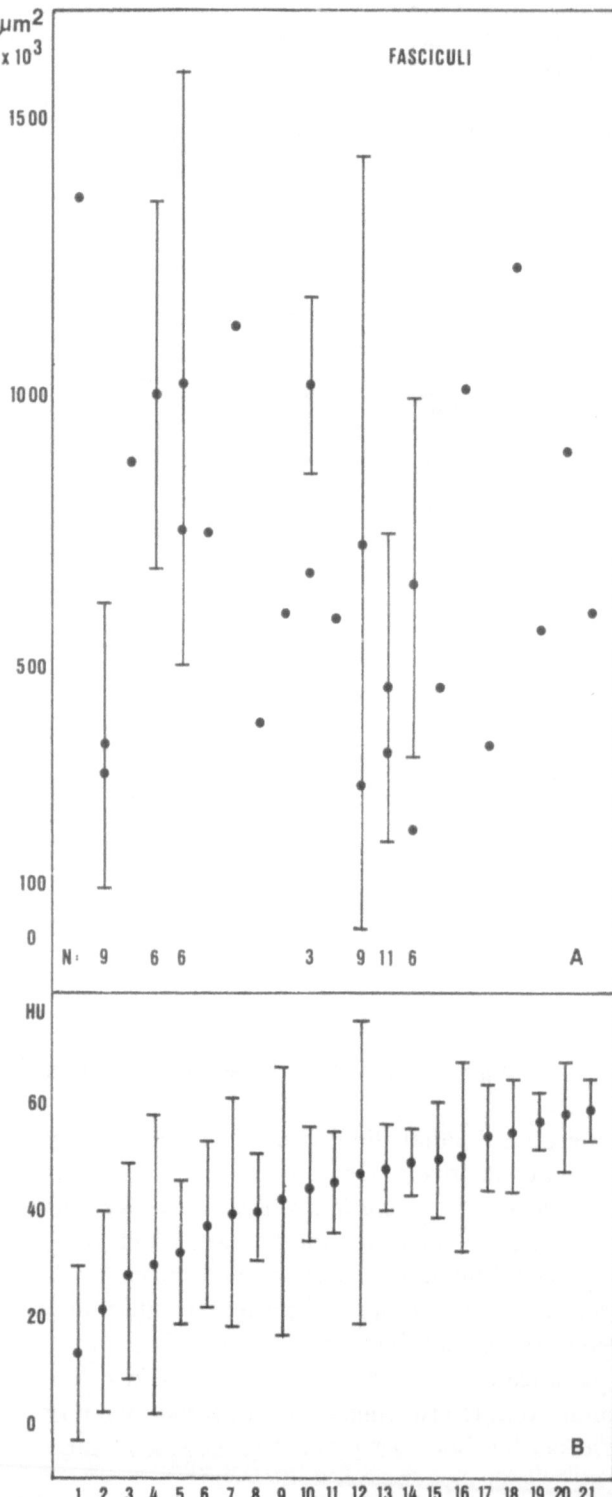

Fig. 8.1 A, B. Correlation between the cross section (in µm²) of muscular fasciculi in 21 biopsies of m. quadriceps femoris **A** compared to density measurements (Hounsfield units, *HU*) in the same patients **B.** Numbers under bar graphs indicate the number of fasciculi included. Each bar graph represents the mean ±1 SD of the mean

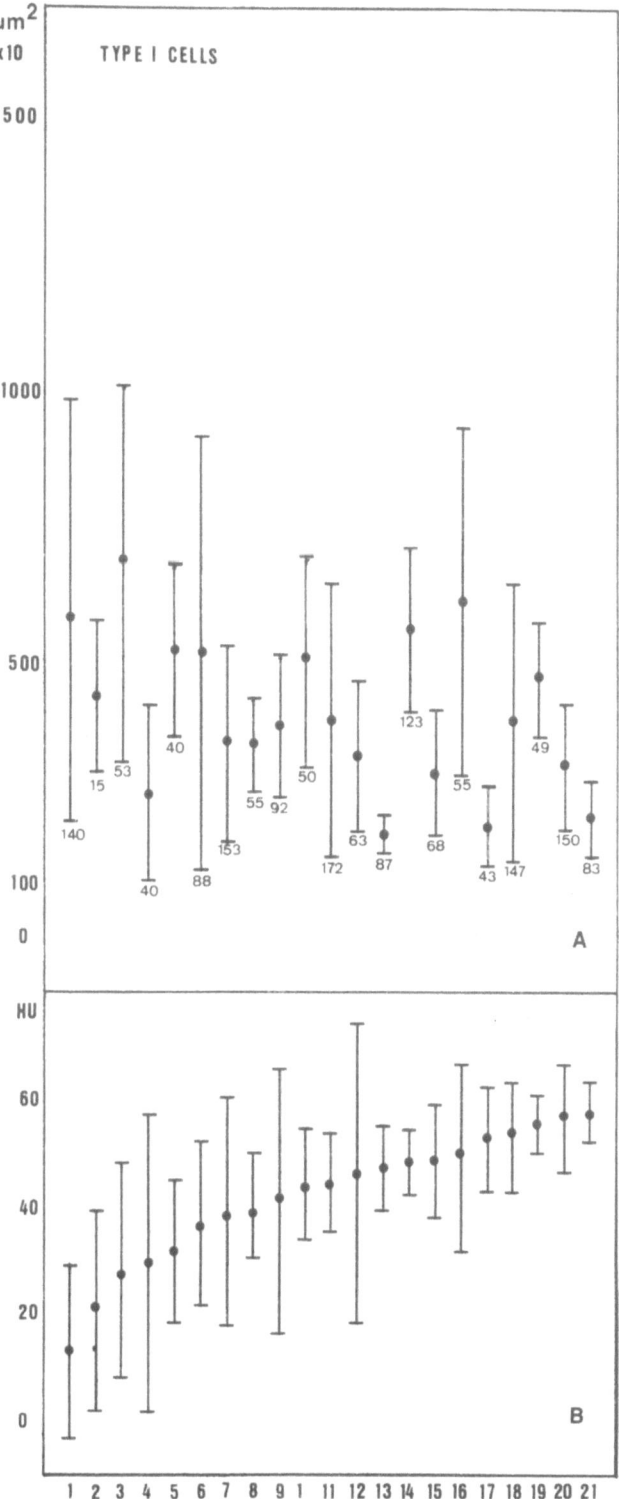

Fig. 8.2 A, B. Correlation between the cross section (in μm²) of type I cells **A** and density measurements **B.** The bar graphs in **A** represent the mean surface area ±1 SD of the mean. Under each bar graph the number of cells measured is mentioned

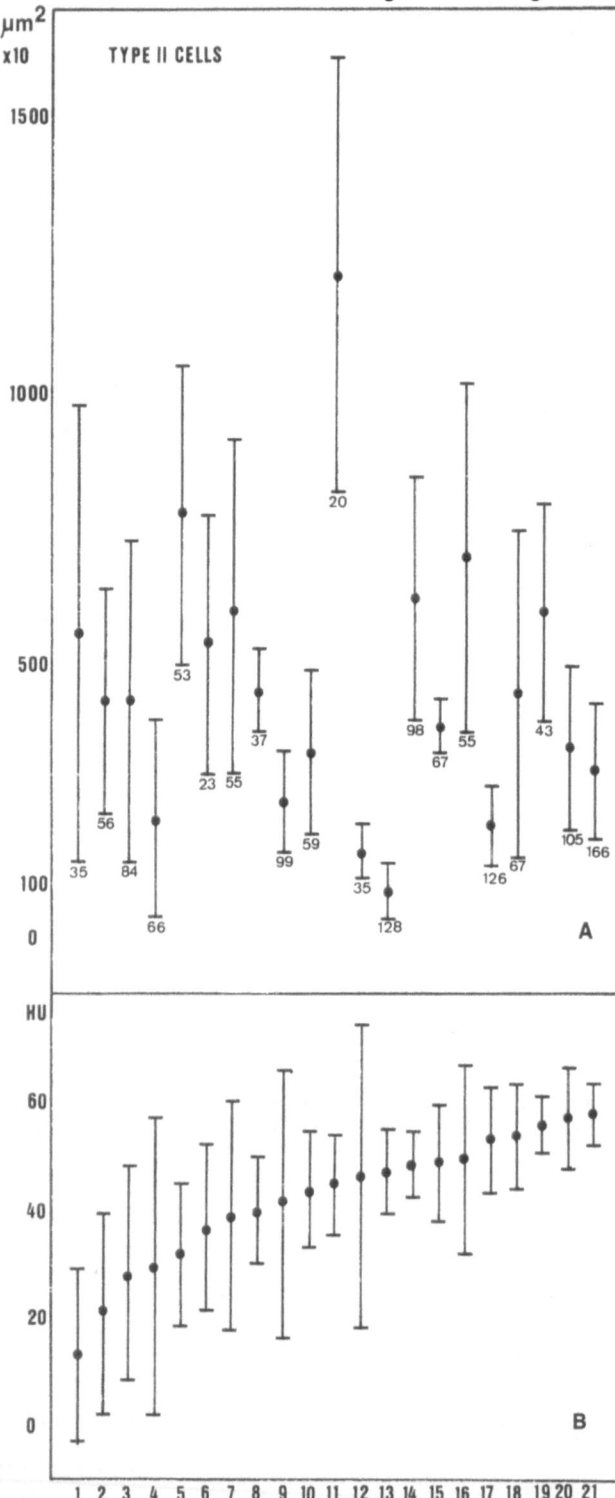

Fig. 8.3 A, B. Correlation between the cross section (in μm^2) of type II cells **A** and density measurements **B.** The bar graphs in **A** represent the mean surface area, in μm^2, ± 1 SD of the mean. Under each bar graph the number of cells measured is mentioned

A normal density measurement is certainly no proof that the measured muscle cells in the region of interest are healthy, just as a normal ECG does not exclude a myocardial infarction, or a normal EEG, epilepsy. We want to illustrate this point further in Figs. 8.4 and 8.5. Figure 8.4 shows a CT scan of the thigh muscles of a 16-year-old girl with a mitochondria-lipid-glycogen (MLG) disease of muscle as described by JERUSALEM et al. (1973) and DI DONATO et al. (1978). The density measurements and the general morphology of the right m. vastus lateralis can be considered normal, but a muscular biopsy taken from this muscle is severely abnormal, as can be seen in Fig. 8.5.

8.2 Correlations Between CT Scanning and EMG

Needle electromyography has undoubtedly established itself as one of the major techniques in the diagnosis of neuromuscular diseases, although some controversy exists as to the significance of certain terms used, such as "neurogenic" and "myogenic" (W. K. ENGEL 1977).

In clincial practice, however, many physicians have been confronted with EMG results which either were reported as within normal limits in cases of well-established neuromuscular disease or failed to detect clinically visible signs, such as fasciculations. Other recordings, on the contrary, show bizarre abnormalities where none were clinically suspected.

In a previous publication (BULCKE et al. 1979b) we have demonstrated that, apart from many other factors which may be involved in such discrepancies between clinical and EMG findings (from the temperature of the examining room to the care with which EMG is carried out), the position of the needle within the various areas of diseased muscle is of great importance.

In a 32-year-old female who was a manifesting carrier of X-linked pseudohypertrophic muscular dystrophy of the Duchenne type, standard needle electrodes (MEDELEC) having an outer diameter of 0.45 mm, a length of 50 mm and a core pick-up area of 0.07 mm^3 were inserted into the muscles under CT control on the video screen. The position of the needles is shown in Figs. 8.6 and 8.7. The potentials derived from these electrodes were amplified and displayed on a MEDELEC MS 6 two-channel electromyograph provided with a fibre optic recording system.

The results of the EMG recordings, all during maximal muscular effort against resistance, are presented in Figs. 8.8–8.10. It can easily be seen that in the most severely infiltrated or atrophied muscles a maximum of EMG changes are found, most characteristic of primary muscular involvement. This finding indicates that in such areas many muscle fibres are still pres-

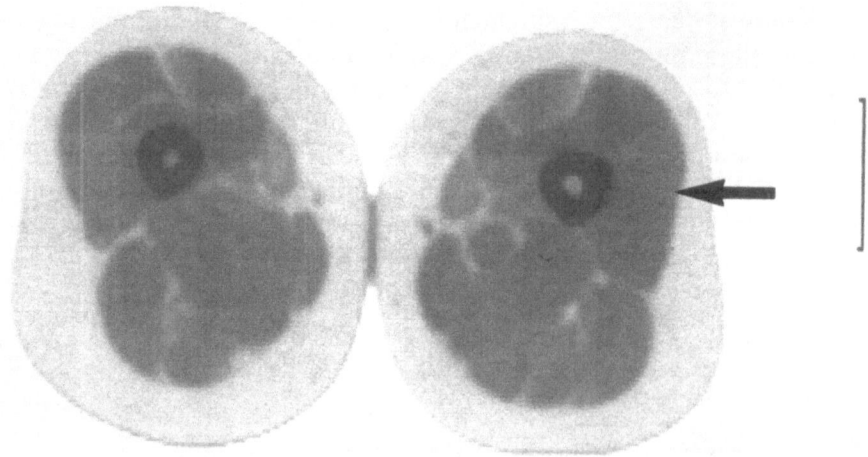

Fig. 8.4

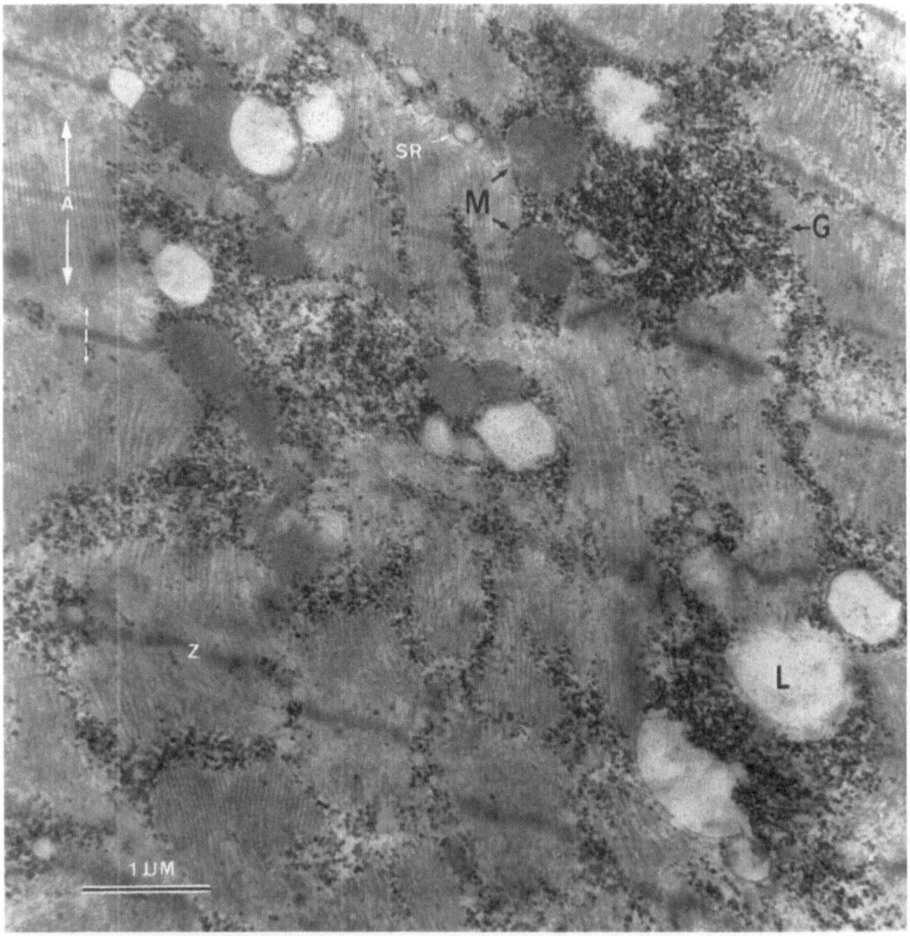

Fig. 8.5

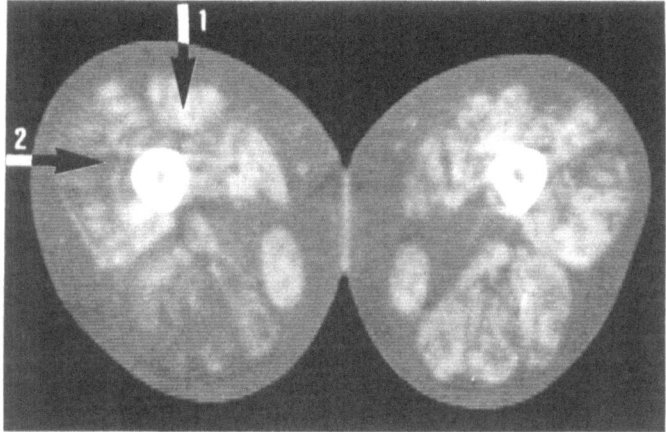

Fig. 8.6. Thigh muscles of a 32-year-old female, a manifesting carrier of Duchenne-type muscular dystrophy. This patient is represented in Fig. 2.4 as carrier III-4. *1*, position of needle number 1 in relatively well-preserved m. rectus femoris; *2*, position of needle 2 in atrophic m. vastus lateralis

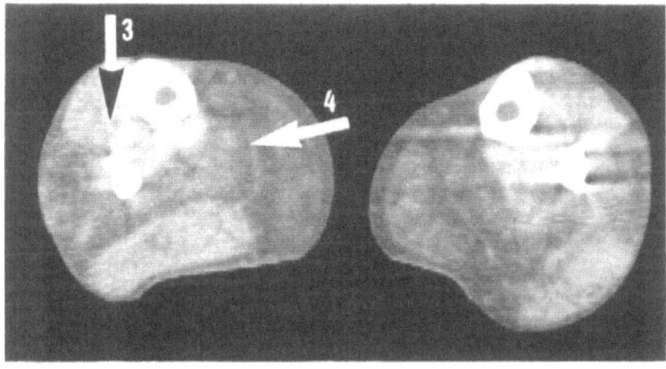

Fig. 8.7. Pseudohypertrophic lower leg muscles of same patient as in Fig. 8.6, *3*, needle inserted into the relatively well-preserved m. tibialis anterior; *4*, needle in atrophic m. gastrocnemius, caput mediale. The tip of the needle reached the fascia between the m. soleus and m. gastrocnemius

Fig. 8.4. Thigh muscles of a 16-year-old girl with a mitochondria-lipid-glycogen disease of muscle as described in the text. Density measurements in the m. quadriceps femoris on both the right and the left side were carried out and found to be normal. A biopsy was taken from the m. quadriceps femoris at the site of the *arrow*. Bar = 5 cm

Fig. 8.5. Electron micrograph (×28500) of the muscle biopsy taken at the site indicated in Fig. 8.4. The biopsy from this area of normal muscular density is very abnormal with accumulation of mitochondria (*M*), proliferation of the cristae, lipid droplets (*L*), and glycogen (*G*), severe disorganization of all sarcomeres with streaming of the Z lines (*Z*) and dilatation of sarcoplasmic reticulum (*SR*). *A*, A band, *I*, I band

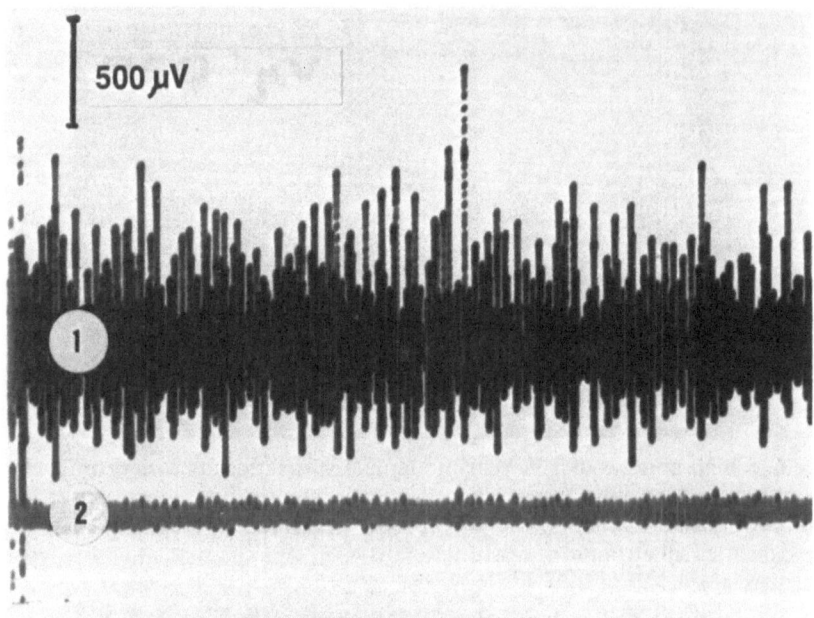

Fig. 8.8. Pattern 1 is recorded from needle 1 in the m. rectus femoris during exten-
sion of the knee. Pattern 2 is taken from the m. vastus lateralis during the same
movement. Both patterns are calibrated at 500 μV and the *horizontal bar* represents 1 s

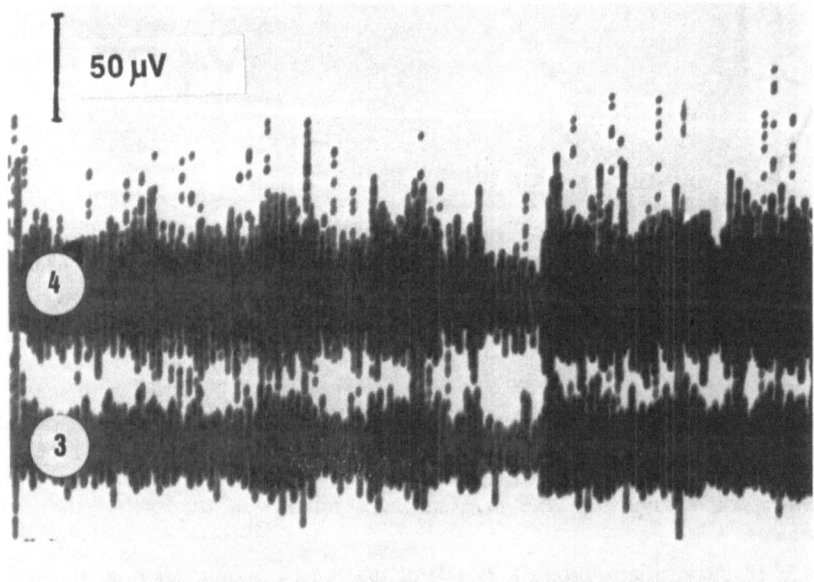

Fig. 8.9. Pattern 4 is obtained from needle 4 in the atrophic m. gastrocnemius, caput
mediale, during plantar flexion of the foot. Pattern 3 is recorded from the m. tibialis
anterior and shows concomitant activity of this muscle during the same movement.
Both recordings are calibrated at 50 μV. The *horizontal bar* represents 1 s

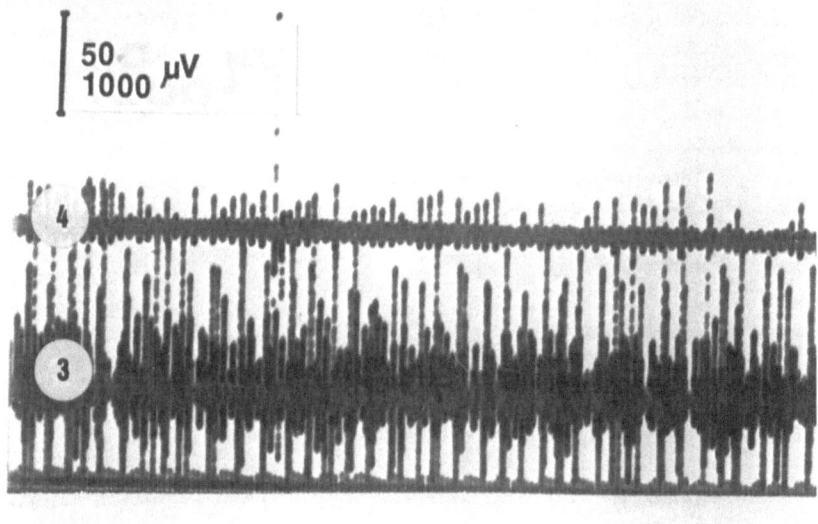

Fig. 8.10. Pattern 3 is recorded from the m. tibialis anterior during dorsiflexion and inversion of the foot, while EMG pattern 4 shows concomitant activity from the m. gastrocnemius. Pattern 4 is calibrated at 50 μV and 3 at 1000 μV. The *horizontal bar* represents 1 s

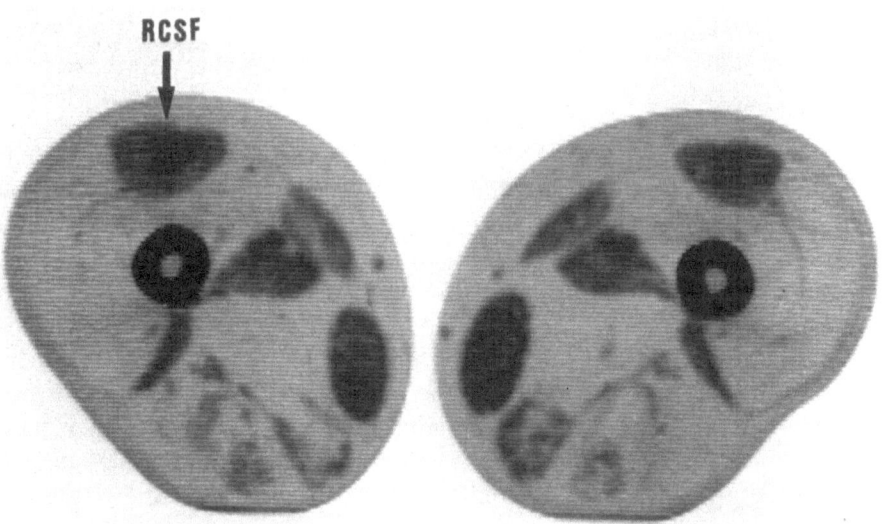

Fig. 8.11. Thigh muscles of a 46-year-old male with a polysaccharide accumulation myopathy as described in the text. By means of single-fibre electromyography, 18 pairs of potentials of motor units were examined in the m. rectus femoris (*RCSF*). The results are summarized in Table 8.3

Table 8.3. Results of selective SFEMG in the right m. rectus femoris

Potential	MCD[a]	Blocking Y/N[b]
1	140.6 +[c]	N
2	88.8 +	N
3	118.4 +	N
4	118.4 +	N
5	540.2 +	Y
6	296.0 +	N
7	74.0 +	N
8	66.6 +	N
9	118.4 +	N
10	118.4 +	N
11	74.0 +	N
12	148.0 +	N
13	148.0 +	N
14	42.92+	N
15	140.6 +	N
16	148.0 +	N
17	222.0 +	N
18	74.0 +	N

Mean MCD: 148.74 ± 114.38 (1 SD)
Fibre density: 2.4

[a] MCD mean of consecutive differences expressed in μs
[b] Y/N, yes or no
[c] +, abnormal value

ent. A typical "myopathic" interference pattern of reduced amplitude is present only where muscle wasting is most evident. The typical example here is the m. gastrocnemius. This means that the territories here examined contain fewer fibres per motor unit, with the total number of motor units remaining normal. The normal recruitment mechanism seems intact, but more motor units are recruited and fire more rapidly than normal for comparable tension. The decreased amplitude has to be explained by a corresponding decrease in amplitude and duration of individual spike potentials. When the loss of functioning muscle fibres progresses further, then even the total number of motor units will decrease, resulting in a pattern of reduced recruitment, while the remaining motor units generate potentials too short and too small to summate adequately. Such a pattern is seen in the m. vastus lateralis.

The patterns in the m. tibialis anterior and m. rectus femoris during full recruitment are almost normal, except for minor changes in the mean action potential duration, the mean inter-spike interval and the range of the absolute refractory period (CARUSO and BUCHTAL 1965). Abnormalities in these muscles could probably be better demonstrated by quantitative EMG (WILLISON 1964, 1966, 1968; ROSE and WILLISON 1968).

A similar experiment was carried out in a 46-year-old male with a myopathy with polysaccharide accumulation (KARPATI et al. 1969; BRUCHER et al. 1982). In Fig. 8.11 the thigh muscles of this patient are shown. Very selective sparing of a limited number of muscles is present, allowing the patient to walk without assistance. Examination of the muscular power of the m. quadriceps reveals a 3-4/5 score according to the MRC (M.R.C. 1943) classification, although only the m. rectus femoris is still present. A single-fibre examination was selectively carried out in this m. rectus femoris. The results of the examination of 18 potential combinations are summarized in Table 8.3. As can be seen, all MCD values which can be considered to be a statistical expression of the stability of the neuromuscular junctions under investigation are abnormal, and the mean value is significantly elevated. The normal value for the m. rectus femoris is 31.0 ± 12.6 (STÅLBERG and TRONDELJ 1979). The mean fibre density is also raised above the normal value of 1.57 ± 0.23 (STÅLBERG and TRONDELJ 1979). These results indicate that the m. rectus femoris seen on CT scanning is certainly not a remnant, a ruin, of the original muscle, but an active entity in which continuous regeneration takes place with sprouting, creating enlarged motor units, very unstable neuromuscular junctions and amazing functional power.

8.3 Correlations Between Muscular Density Measurements and Muscular Power Parameters in m. vastus lateralis

In the same group of patients described in Table 8.2, muscular power parameters in m. quadriceps femoris were measured. Muscular power was graded 0–5 according to the known MRC scale. The results are summarized in Table 8.4. As can be seen, within the narrow range of density measurements important variations can exist in muscular power. The relationship between density measurements and muscular power is poor. It is obvious that the patient shown in Fig. 8.12, with an end-stage of Duchenne muscular dystrophy and very low density values, is inevitably confined to a wheelchair. The patient in Fig. 8.13, however, has almost normal density readings but very poor muscular power (1-3/5) which also confines the patient to a wheelchair, although the morphology of the scan certainly does not suggest this.

In general it seems that patients with selective atrophies and/or compensatory hypertrophy as shown in Figs. 6.22 and 6.23 remain independent much longer than those without these phenomena.

Table 8.4. Correlations between density measurements and muscular power

Case no.	Measurement of density (HU)	Power in m. quadriceps					
		0	1	2	3	4	5
1	14.10 ± 16.24	——————————					
2	21.30 ± 18.27	N. D.					
3	28.30 ± 19.65	—————————					
4	30.10 ± 26.81	——————————					
5	32.50 ± 13.10	———————————————————					
6	38.10 ± 14.98	N. D					
7	40.18 ± 21.16	———————————————————					
8	41.00 ± 8.69	—————————					
9	41.60 ± 24.80	N. D.					
10	44.90 ± 10.25	———————————————————					
11	45.70 ± 8.20	—————————————————					
12	46.60 ± 27.93	N. D.					
13	47.01 ± 7.82	N. D.					
14	49.90 ± 4.40	———————————————————					
15	50.20 ± 10.19	—————————————————					
16	50.50 ± 16.25	—————————					
17	53.93 ± 8.98	N. D.					
18	54.17 ± 8.98	—————————————————					
19	56.74 ± 5.13	N. D.					
20	57.51 ± 9.83	N. D.					
21	59.36 ± 4.65	———————————————————					

N. D., Not determined

Fig. 8.12 A–C. This 12-year-old boy with Duchenne muscular dystrophy (see Fig. 2.4, IV-4) has severe atrophy of all muscles. He is either wheelchair-bound or bed-ridden. Bar = 5 cm

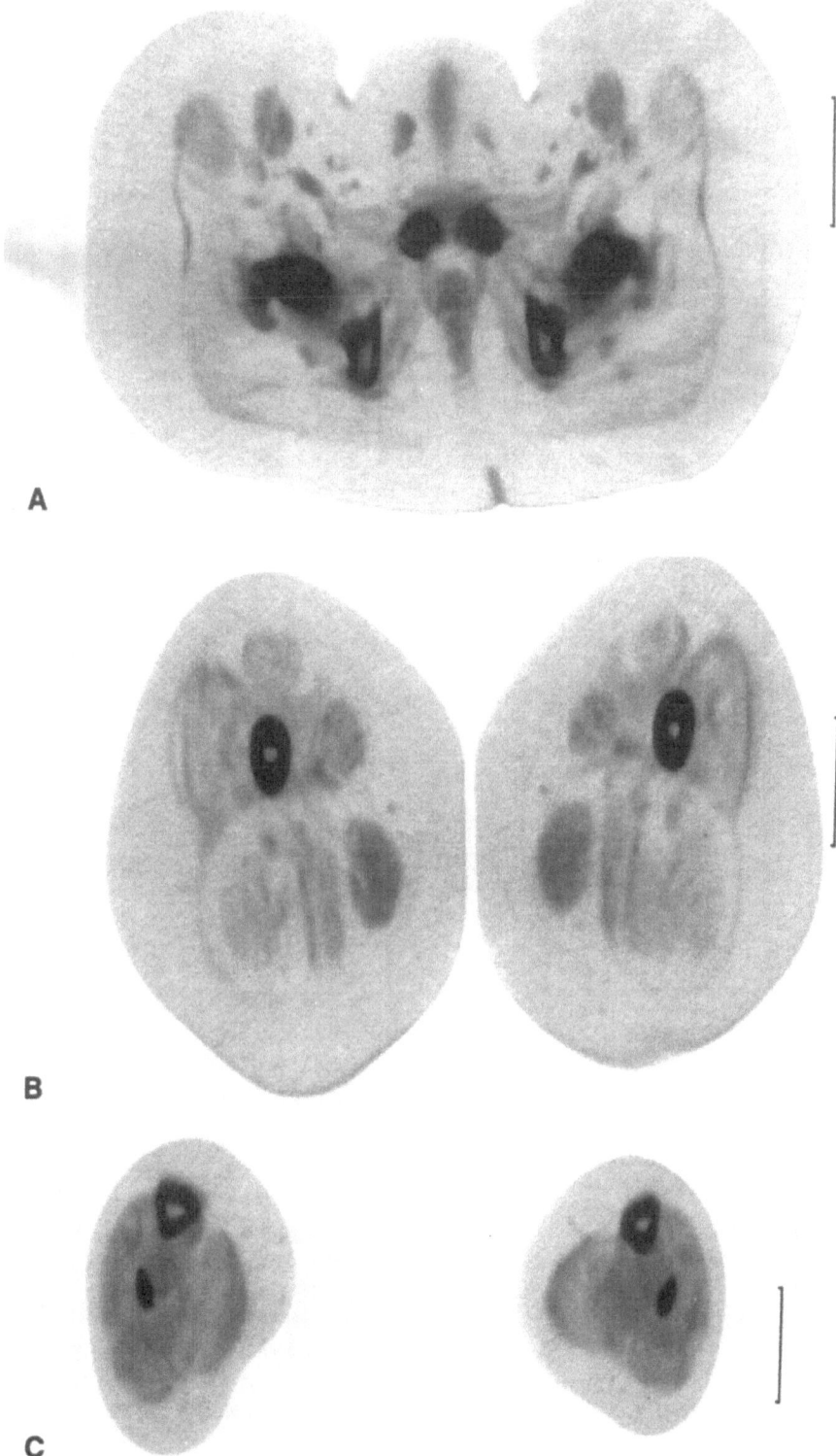

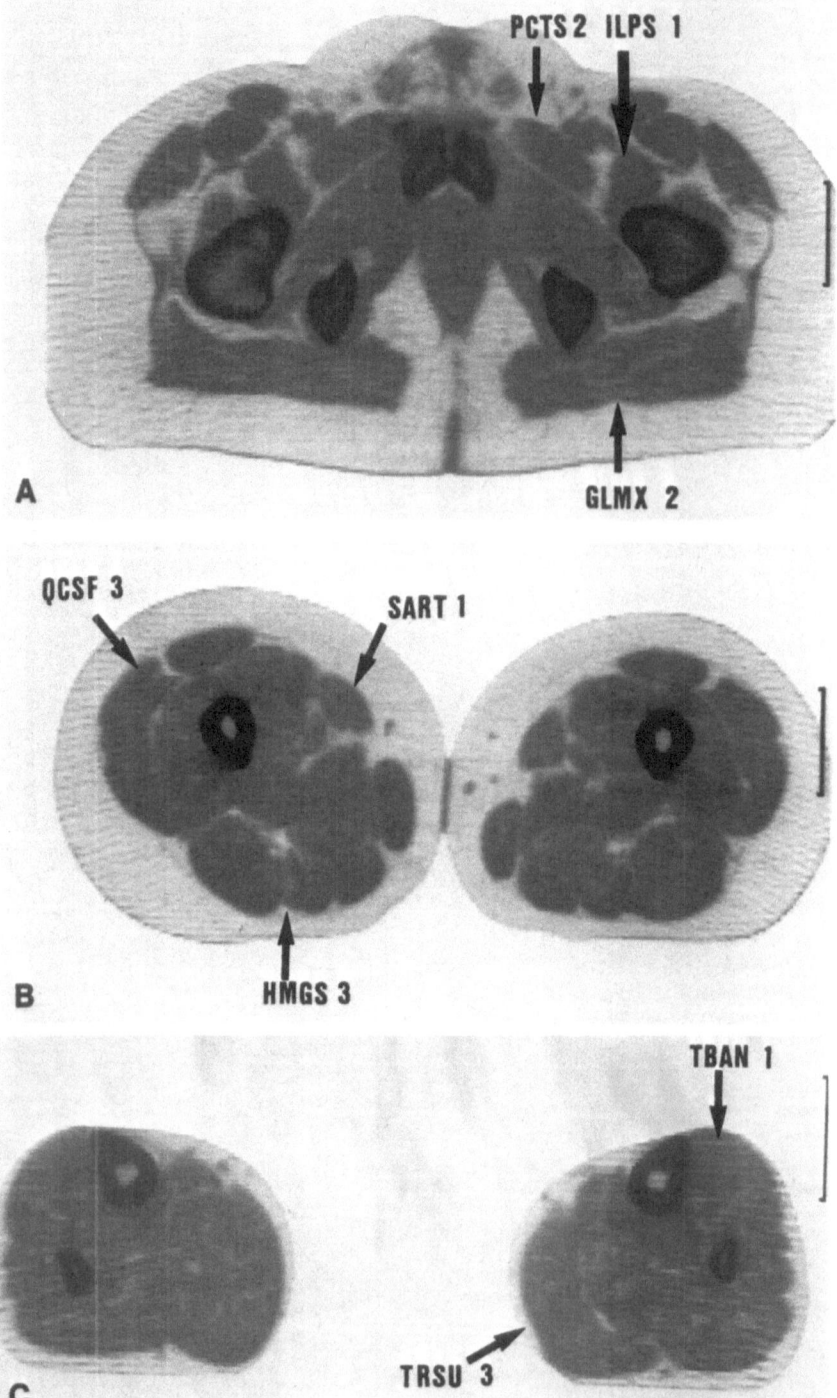

Fig. 8.13. A Pelvic muscles, **B** thigh muscles and **C** lower leg muscles of a 42-year-old male with an autosomal recessive myopathy of unknown aetiology. Muscular density is normal. Muscular power values of m. iliopsoas (*ILPS*), m. gluteus maximus (*GLMX*), m. pectineus (*PCTS*), m. sartorius (*SART*), hamstrings (*HMGS*), m. quadriceps femoris (*QCSF*), m. tibialis anterior (*TBAN*) and m. triceps surae (*TRSU*) are indicated next to the muscle names. Bar = 5 cm

References

Abramson AS (1948) Bone disturbances in injuries to spinal cord and cauda equina (paraplegia) their prevention by ambulation. J Bone Joint Surg [Am] 30: 982–987

Ackerman LV (1958) Extra-osseous localised non-neoplastic bone and carthilago formation (so-called myositis ossificans). J Bone Joint Surg [Am] 40:279–298

Adams RD (1975) Diseases of muscle. A study in pathology, 3rd edn. Harper & Row

Adrian RH, Marshall MW (1976) Action potentials reconstructed in normal and myotonic muscle fibres. J Physiol (Lond) 258:125–143

Akin RA, Keller AJ, Walters PJ (1975) Myositis ossificans progressiva: a diagnostic problem. J Oral Surg 33:611–615

Alfidi RD, Haaga J, Weinstein M, de Groot J (1977) Computed tomography of the human body. An atlas of normal anatomy. Mosby, St Louis

Allen EP, Calder HW (1940) Soft tissue radiography. Br J Radiol 13:422–427

Anderson JE (1978) Grant's atlas of anatomy, 7th edn. Williams & Wilkins, Baltimore

Barbosa J, Nuttal FQ, Kennedy W, Goetz F (1974) Plasma insulin in patients with myotonic dystrophy. Medicine (Baltimore) 53:307–323

Barchi RL (1975) Myotonia: an evaluation of the chloride hypothesis. Arch Neurol 32:175–180

Barucha EP, Pandya SS, Dastur DK (1972) Arthrogryposis multiplex congenita: Part 1: Clinical and electromyographic aspects. J Neurol Neurosurg Psychiatry 35:425–434

Batten FE, Gibb HP (1909) Myotonia atrophica. Brain 32:187–205

Becker PE (1962) Two new families of benign sex-linked recessive muscular dystrophy. Rev Can Biol 21:551–566

Becker PE (1977) Syndromes associated with myotonia: clinical – genetic classification. In: Rowland LP (ed) Pathogenesis of human muscular dystrophies, Excerpta Medica, New York, pp 699–703

Becker PE, Kiener F (1955) Eine neue X-chromosomale Muskeldystrophie. Arch Psychiatr Nervenkr 193:427–448

Bellina CR, Brarichi R, Bombardieri S, Feri C, Mariani G, Muratorio A, Rossi B (1978) Quantitative evaluation of ^{99m}Tc-pyrophosphate muscle uptake in patients with inflammatory and noninflammatory muscle diseases. J Nucl Med Allied Sci 22:89–96

Bellon EM, Miraldi FD, Wiesen EJ (1979) Performance evaluation of computed tomography scanners using a phantom model. AJR 132:345–352

Benassy J (1966) Ossification and fracture healing in paraplegia and brain injuries. Proc Ann Clin Spinal Cord Inj Conf 15:55–70

Berger PE, Kuhn JP (1978) Computed tomography of tumors of the muskuloskelet-al system in children: clinical applications. Radiology 127:171–176

Bergsma D (ed) (1979) Birth defects compendium. The national foundation – March of Dimes. MacMillan, London Bazingstoke

Bethlem J (1977) Myopathies. Elsevier/North-Holland Biomedical Press, Amsterdam New York Oxford

Betten MG, Bilchik RC, Smith ME (1971) Pigmentary retinopathy of myotonic dystrophy. Am J Ophtalmol 72:720–723

Blahd WD, Lederer M, Cassen B (1967) The significance of decreased body potassium concentration in patients with muscular dystrophy and nondystrophic relatives. N Engl J Med 276:1349–1352

Blyth H, Carter CO, Dubowitz V, Emery AEH, Gavin J, Johnston HA, McKusick VA, Sanger R, Tippett P (1965) Duchenne's muscular dystrophy and the Xg blood groups: a search for linkage. J Med Genet 2:157–160

Boag JW (1973) Xeroradiography. Phys Med Biol 18:3–37

Bodensteiner JG, Engel AG (1978) Intracellular calcium accumulation in Duchenne dystrophy and other myopathies: A study of 567,000 muscle fibers in 114 biopsies. Neurology (Minneap) 28:439–446

Bosma JF, Brodie OR (1969) Cineradiographic demonstration of pharyngeal area myotonia in myotonic dystrophy patients. Radiology 92:104–109

Bossen EH, Shelburne JD, Verkauf BS (1974) Respiratory muscle involvement in infantile myotonic dystrophy. Arch Pathol 97:250–252

Bourne GH (ed) (1973a) The structure and function of muscle, vol I: Structure. Part 1. Academic Press, New York London

Bourne GH (ed) (1973b) The structure and function of muscle, vol II: Structure. Part 2. Academic Press, New York London

Bourne GH (ed) (1973c) The structure and function of muscle, vol III: Physiology and biochemistry. Academic Press, New York London

Bourne GH (ed) (1973d) The structure and function of muscle, vol IV: Pharmacology and disease. Academic Press, New York London

Bradley WG, Jones MZ, Mussini J-M, Fawcett PRW (1978) Becker-type muscular dystrophy. Muscle Nerve 1:111–132

Bree RL, Green B, Keiller DL, Genet EF (1976) Medial deviation of the ureters secondary to psoas muscle hypertrophy. Radiology 188:691–695

Brill DR (1981) Radionuclide imaging of nonneoplastic soft tissue disorders. Semin Nucl Med 11:277–288

Brodal A (1981) Neurological anatomy in relation to clinical medicine. Oxford University Press, New York Oxford. 3rd edn. pp 1–1053

Brooke MH, Kaiser KK (1970) Muscle fibre types: How many and what kind? Arch Neurol 23:369–379

Brown M, Swift TR, Spies SM (1976) Radioisotope scanning in inflammatory muscle disease. Neurology (Minneap) 26:517–520

Brucher J-M, Tassin S, de Barsy T, Dom R, Bulcke J (1982) Muscle polysaccharidosis: A rare disease. (Submitted for publication)

Budin JA, Feldman F (1975) Soft tissue calcifications in systemic lupus erythematosus. AJR 124:358–364

Bulcke JA, Termote J-L, Palmers Y, Crolla D (1979a) Computed tomography of the human skeletal muscular system. Neuroradiology 17:127–136

Bulcke JA, de Meirsman J, Termote J-L (1979b) The influence of skeletal muscle atrophy on needle electromyography. As demonstrated by computed tomography. Electromyogr Clin Neurophysiol 19:269–279

Bulcke JA, Crolla D, Termote J-L, Baert A, Palmers Y, van den Bergh R (1981) Computed tomography of muscle. Muscle Nerve 4:67–72

Burke RE, Levine DM, Zajac FE, Tsairis P, Engel WK (1971) Mammalian motor units: physiological–histochemical correlation in three types in cat gastrocnemius. Science 174:709–712

Busch WA, Stromer MH, Goll DE, Suzuki A (1972) Ca^{2+}-specific removal of Z lines from rabbit skeletal muscle. J Cell Biol 52:367–381

Buya LM, Parkey RW, Dees JH, Stokeley EM, Harris RA, Bonte FJ, Willerson JT (1975) Morphologic correlates of technetium-99m stannous pyrophosphate imaging of acute myocardial infarcts in dogs. Circulation 52:596–607

Campbell WL, Feldman F (1975) Bone and soft tissue abnormalities of the upper extremity in diabetes mellitus. AJR 124:7–16

Cao A, Chianchetti C, Calisti L, de Virgilis S, Ferreli A, Tangheroni W (1978) Schwartz-Jampel syndrome. Clinical, electrophysiological and histopathological study of a severe variant. J Neurol Sci 35:175–181

Carroll JE, Zwillich CW, Weil JV (1977) Ventilatory response in myotonic dystrophy. Neurology (Minneap) 27:1125–1128

Caruso D, Buchtal F (1965) Refractory period of muscle and findings in relatives of patients with muscular dystrophy. Brain 88:29–50

Caughey JE (1952) Radiological changes in skull in dystrophia myotonica. Brit Med J 1:137–139

Caughey JE, Myrianthopoulos NC (1963) Dystrophia myotonica and related disorders. Thomas, Springfield

Chang SF (1978) Pear-shaped bladder caused by large iliopsoas muscles. Radiology 128:349–350

Chassevent J, Sauvegrain J, Besson-Leaud M, Kalifa G (1978) Myotonic dystrophy (Steinert's disease) in the neonate. Radiology 127:747–749

Coërs C, Desmedt JE (1959) Mise en evidence d'une malformation de la jonction neuromusculaire dans la myasthénie. Acta Neurol Belg 59:539–561

Coërs C, Telermann-Toppet N (1979) Differential diagnosis of limb-girdle muscular dystrophy and spinal muscular atrophy. Neurology (Minneap) 29:957–972

Collatos TC, Edgerton VR, Smith JL, Botterman BR (1977) Contractile properties and fibre type compositions of flexors and extensors of elbow joint in cat: Implications for motor control. J Neurophysiol 40:1292–1300

Collins JD, Pagani JJ (1978) Extrathoracic musculature mimicking pleural lesions. Radiology 129:21–22

Costill DL, Tink WJ, Pollock ML (1976) Skeletal muscle enzymes and fibre composition in male and female track athletes. J Appl Physiol 40:149–154

Culebras A (1977) Absence of sleep-related growth hormone elevations in myotonic dystrophy. Neurology (Minneap) 27:165–167

Curshmann H (1912) Über familiäre atrophische Myotonie. Dtsch Z Nervenheilkd 45:161–197

Damansky M (1961) Heterotopic ossification in paraplegia – a clinical study. J Bone Joint Surg [Br] 43:286–299

Dark AJ, Streeten BW (1977) Ultrastructural study of cataract in myotonia dystrophica. Am J Ophthalm 84:666–674

DeBacker M, Bergmann P, Perissino A, Gottignies P, Kahn RJ (1976) Respiratory failure and cardiac disturbances in myotonic dystrophy. Europ J Intens Care Med 2:63–67

Delwaide PA, Delwaide PJ, Penders CA (1972) Isotope studies of body composition in neuromuscular diseases. J Neurol Sci 15:339–349

Desai A, Eymontt M, Alavi A, Schaffer B, Dalinka MK (1972) ^{99m}Tc-MDP uptake in nonosseous lesions. Radiology 135:181–184

Di Chiro G, Nelson KB (1965) Soft tissue radiography of the extremities in neuromuscular disease with histological correlations. Acta Radiol [Diagn] (Stockh) 3:65–88

Di Donato S, Cornelis F, Balestrini MR, Bertagnolio B, Peluchetti D (1978) Mitochondria-lipid-glycogen myopathy, hyperlactacidemia and carnitine deficiency. Neurology (Minneap) 28:1110–1116

Doust DB, Ting YM (1974) Xeroradiology of the larynx. Radiology 110:727–730

Dubowitz V (1969) The floppy infant. Heinemann, London; Lippincott, Philadelphia (Clinics in developmental medicine, no 31)

Dubowitz V, Brooke MH (1973) Muscle biopsy: a modern approach. Saunders, London Philadelphia Toronto

Duncan CJ (1978) Role of intracellular calcium in promoting muscle damage: a strategy for controlling the dystrophic condition. Experientia 34:1531–1535

Eaton WL, Conkling WS, Daeschner CW (1957) Early myositis ossificans progressiva occurring in homozygotic twins. A clinical and pathologic study. J Pediatr 50:591–598

Edgerton UR, Smith JL, Simpson DR (1975) Muscle fibre type population of human leg muscles. Histochem J 7:259–269

Edstrom L (1968) Histochemical changes in upper motor lesions, parkinsonism and disuse. Differential effect on white and red muscle fibers. Experientia 24:916–918

Edstrom L, Ekblom B (1972) Differences in sizes of red and white muscle fibres in vastus lateralis of musculus quadriceps femoris of normal individuals and athletes. Relation to physical performance. Scand J Clin Lab Invest 30:175–181

Edstrom L, Nystrom B (1969) Histochemical types and sizes of fibres in normal human muscles. Acta Physiol Scand 45:257–269

Ellis M, Frank HG (1966) Myositis ossificans traumatica: with special reference to the quadriceps femoris muscle. J Trauma 6:724–738

Emery AEH (1966) Genetic linkage between the loci for colour blindness and Duchenne-type muscular dystrophy. J Med Genet 3:92–95

Emery AEH, Dreifuss FE (1966) Unusual type of benign X-linked muscular dystrophy. J Neurol Neurosurg Psychiatry 29:338–342

Emery AEH, Skinner R (1976) Clinical studies in benign (Becker type) X-linked muscular dystrophy. Clin Genet 10:189–201

Emery AEH, Clarck ER, Simon S, Taylor JL (1967) Detection of carriers of benign X-linked muscular dystrophy. Br Med J 4:522–523

Emery AEH, Smith CAB, Sanger R (1969) The linkage relations of the loci for benign (Becker type) X-borne muscular dystrophy, colour blindness and the Xg blood groups. Ann Hum Genet 32:261–269

Engel AG (1979) Myasthenia gravis. In: Vinken PJ, Bruyn GW (eds) Handbook of clinical neurology, vol 41. North-Holland, Amsterdam New York Oxford, pp 95–145

Engel AG, Lambert EH, Howard FM (1977a) Immune complexes (Igb and C_3) at the motor end-plate in myasthenia gravis. Ultrastructural and light microscopic localisation and electrophysiological correlations. Mayo Clin Proc 52:267–280

Engel AG, Lindstrom JM, Lambert EH, Lennon VA (1977b) Ultrastructural localisation of the acetylcholine receptor in myasthenia gravis and in its experimental autoimmune model. Neurology (Minneap) 27:307–315

Engel WK (1977) Integrative histochemical approach to the defect in Duchenne muscular dystrophy. In: Rowland LP (ed) Pathogenesis of human muscular dystrophies. Excerpta Medica, Amsterdam, pp 227–309

Enzmann D, Marshall WH, Rosenthal AR, Kris JP (1976) Computed tomography in Graves' ophtalmopathy. Radiology 118:615–620

Eulenburg A (1886) Über eine familiäre, durch 6 Generationen verfolgbare Form congenitaler Paramyotonie. Neurol Zentralbl 5:265–272

Feinstein B, Lindegård B, Nyman E, Wohlfart G (1955) Morphologic studies of motor units in normal human muscles. Acta Anat (Basel) 23:127–142

Festoff BW, Moore WV (1979) Evaluation of the insulin receptor in myotonic dystrophy. Ann Neurol 6:60–65

Filippi G (1971) Benign muscular dystrophy, Becker type. Birth Defects 72:110–112

Fisher RL, Johnstone WT, Fisher WH, Goldkamp OG (1970) Arthrogryposis multiplex congenita: A clinical investigation. J Pediatr 76:255–261

Frantzell A (1951) Soft tissue radiography. Acta Radiol [Suppl] (Stockh) 85

Frantzell A, Ingelmark BE (1951) Occurrence and distribution of fat in human muscles at various age levels. A morphologic and roentgenologic examination. Upsala läkaref förh 56:59–87

Frantzell A, Hagberg B, Söderhjelm L (1952) Werdnig-Hoffmann's progressive muscular atrophy. Creatine excretion following vitamin E treatment and muscle radiography. Upsala läkaref förh 56:209–223

Fredericks EJ, Russmann BS (1979) Bedside evaluation of large motor units in childhood spinal muscular atrophy. Neurology (Minneap) 29:398–400

Frischknecht W, Bianchi L, Pilleri G (1960) Familial arthrogryposis complex congenita. Neuroarthromyodysplasia congenita. Helv Paediat Acta 15:259–279

Gaffney BJ, Drachman DB, Lin DC, Tennekoon G (1980) Spin-label studies of erythrocytes in myotonic dystrophy. No increase in membrane fluidity. Neurology (NY) 30:272–276

Gambarelli J, Guérinel G, Chevrot L, Mattei M (1977) Coupes sériées du corps humain. Anatomie-radiologie-scanner. Springer, Berlin Heidelberg New York

Gamsu G, Mark AS, Webb WR (1981) Computed tomography of the normal larynx during quiet breathing and phonation. J Comput Assist Tomogr 5:353–360

Gay BB Jr, Kuhn JP (1976) A syndrome of widened medullary cavities of bone, aortic calcification, abnormal dentition and muscular weakness (The Singleton-Merten syndrome). Radiology 118:389–395

Gillain PMS, Heaf PJD, Kaufman L, Lucas BGB (1964) Respiration in dystrophia myotonica. Thorax 19:112–120

Gilmartin D (1979) The serratus anterior muscle on chest radiographs. Radiology 131:629–635

Goldsmith BM, Gruemer H-D, Hawley RJ, Pickard NA, Verrill HL, Nance WE, Miller G, Crawford RG (1980) The contribution of assays of lymphocyte capping and creatine kinase to detection of the Becker-type dystrophy trait. Clin Chem 26:754–759

Gollnick PD, Armstrong RB, Saubert IV CW, Piehl K, Saltin B (1972) Enzyme activity and fibre type composition in skeletal muscle of untrained and trained men. J Appl Physiol 33:312–319

Gollnick PD, Armstrong RB, Saltin B, Saubert IV CW, Sembrowich WL, Shepherd RE (1973) Effect of training on enzyme activity and fiber composition of human skeletal muscle. J Appl Physiol 34:107–111

Gollnick PD, Sjödin B, Karlsson J, Jansson E, Saltin B (1974) Human soleus muscle: a comparison of fibre composition and enzyme activities with other leg muscles. Pfluegers Arch 348:247–255

Grabbe E, Heller M, Böcker W (1979) Computed tomography in soft tissue sarcomas. ROEFO 131:372–378

Greig DN (1977) Family in which Duchenne's muscular dystrophy and protan colour blindness are segregating. J Med Genet 14:130–132

Griggs RC, Davis RJ, Anderson DC, Dove JI (1975) Cardiac conduction in myotonic dystrophy. Am J Med 59:37–42

Guilleminault C (1978) Baclofen trial in six myotonic dystrophy patients. Acta Neurol Scand 57:232–238

Habener JF, Potts JT Jr (1978a) Biosynthesis of parathyroid hormone (Part 1). N' Engl J Med 299:580–585

Habener JF, Potts JT Jr (1978b) Biosynthesis of parathyroid hormone (Part 2). N Engl J Med 299:635–644

Häggmark T, Jansson E, Svane B (1978) Cross-sectional area of thigh muscle in man measured by computed tomography. Scand J Clin Lab Invest 38:355–360

Harle TS, Hevezi JM, Rogers LF, Martin JE, Bao-Shang Jing (1975) Xerotomography of the tracheobroncheal tree. AJR 124:353–357

Harper PS (1975a) Congenital myotonic dystrophy in Britain. I. Clinical aspects. Arch Dis Child 50:505–513

Harper PS (1975b) Congenital myotonic dystrophy in Britain. II. Genetic basis. Arch Dis Child 50:514–521

Harper PS (1979) Myotonic dystrophy. Saunders, Philadelphia London Toronto

Hauser SL, Wener HL, Bresnan MJ, Ault KA (1979) Lymphocyte capping in muscular dystrophy. Neurology (Minneap) 29:1419–1421

Hausmanowa-Petrusewicz I, Borkowska J (1978) Intrafamilial variability of X-linked progressive muscular dystrophy. Mild and acute form of X-linked muscular dystrophy in the same family. J Neurol 218:43–50

Haussler MR, McCain TA (1977) Basic and clinical concepts related to vitamin D metabolism and action. N Engl J Med 297:974–983

Hermann GH, Rose JS (1979) Computed tomography in bone and soft tissue pathology of the extremities. J Comput Assist Tomogr 3:58–66

Hounsfield GN (1976) Picture quality of computed tomography. AJR 127:3–9

Hounsfield GN (1978) Potential uses of more accurate C.T. absorption values by filtering. AJR 131:103–106

Hounsfield GN (1980) Computed medical imaging. Nobel lecture, December 8, 1979. J Comput Assist Tomogr 4:665–674

Houten R ten (1979) Limb-girdle muscular dystrophy? Medical dissertation, University of Amsterdam

Ingelmark BE, Helander E (1951) The action of castration and inactivity on the fat content of striated muscle. Upsala läkaref förh 56:95–99

Jeffrey RB, Callen PW, Federle MP (1980) Computed tomography of psoas abscess. J Comput Assist Tomogr 4:639–641

Jennekens FG, Tomlinson BE, Walton JN (1971) Data on the distribution of fibre types in five human limb muscles: an autopsy study. J Neurol Sci 14:245–257

Jerusalem F (1979) Muskelerkrankungen. Klinik-Therapie-Pathologie. Thieme, Stuttgart

Jerusalem F, Angelini C, Engel AG, Groover RV (1973) Mitochondria-lipid-glycogen (MLG) disease of muscle. A morphologically regressive congenital myopathy. Arch Neurol 29:162–169

Jing B-S (1974) The pharynx and larynx: roentgenographic technique. Semin Roentgenol 9:259–265

Johnson MA, Polgar J, Weightman D, Appleton D (1973) Data on the distribution of fibre types in thirty-six human muscles. An autopsy study. J Neurol Sci 18:111–129

Jones BV, Ward MW (1980) Myositis ossificans in the biceps femoris muscles causing sciatic nerve palsy. A case report. J Bone Joint Surg [Br] 62:506–507

Josephson ME, Caracta AR, Gallagher JJ, Damato AN (1973) Site of conduction disturbances in a family with myotonic dystrophy. Am J Cardiol 32:114–118

Kalisher L (1975) Xeroradiography of axillary lymph node disease. Radiology 115:67–71

Karpati G (1977) A review of the morphologic features and consequences of muscle cell necrosis in Duchenne disease: clues to the pathogenesis. Excerpta Med Int Congr Ser 343:117–131

Karpati G, Carpenter S, Wolfe LS, Sherwin A (1969) A peculiar polysaccharide accumulation in muscle in a case of cardioskeletal myopathy. Neurology (Minneap) 19:553–564

Keats TE (1978) Post-injection calcification of the deltoid muscle. J Can Assoc Radiol 29:165–166

Keens TG, Ianuzzo LD (1979) Development of fatigue resistant muscle fibres in human ventilatory muscles. Am Rev Respir Dis 119:139–141

Kewalramani LS (1977) Ectopic ossification. Am J Phys Med 56:99–121

Khan MA, Khan N (1978) Statistical analysis of muscle fibre types from human skeletal muscles. Anat Anz 144:246–256

Klein D (1958) La dystrophie myotonique (Steinert) et la myotonie congénitale (Thomsen) en Suisse. Etude clinique, génétique et géographique. J Genet Hum 7:1–328

Kohaus H, Peters P, Strunk E (1980) Iliopsoas muscle tear. Symptoms and differential diagnosis of an uncommon injury. Unfallheilkunde 83:127–129

Korobkin M (ed) (1978) Computed tomography, ultrasound and X-ray: an integrated approach. University of California Press, Berkeley London

Kossmann RJ, Peterson DC, Andrews HL (1965) Studies in neuro-muscular disease: total body potassium in muscular dystrophy and related diseases. Neurology (Minneap) 15:855–865

Krishnamurthy GT, Huebotter RJ, Walsh CF, Taylor JR, Kehr MD, Tubis M, Blahd WH (1975) Kinetics of ^{99m}Tc-labeled pyrophosphate and polyphosphate in man. J Nucl Med 16:109–115

Kuhn E (1979) Muskeldystrophie: Duchenne- und Becker-Kiener Typ. Dtsch Med Wochenschr 51:1817–1820

Kühn E, Fiehn W (1978) Erhöhte Insulin-Sekretion bei myotonia dystrophica. Fortschr Med 96:577–580

Kugelberg EA, Welander M (1956) Heredofamilial juvenile muscular atrophy simulating muscular dystrophy. Arch Neurol Psychiatry 75:500–509

Kwicienski H (1980) Treatment of myotonic dystrophy with acetazolamide. J Neurol 222:261–264

Larsen B, Johnson G, Van Loghem E, Marshall WH, Neuton RM, Pryse-Phillips W, Skanes V (1980) Immunoglobulin concentration and Gm allotypes in a family with thirty-three cases of myotonic dystrophy. Clin Genet 18:13–19

Larsson L, Sjodin B, Karlsson J (1978) Histochemical and biochemical changes in human skeletal muscle with age in sedentary males, age 22–65 years. Acta Physiol Scand 103:31–39

Latchaw RE, Gold LHA, Moore JS Jr, Payne JT (1977) The nonspecificity of absorption in the differentiation of solid tumor and cystic lesions. Radiology 125:141–144

Ledley RS, Huang HK, Mazziotta JC (1977) Cross-sectional anatomy. An atlas for computerized tomography. Williams & Wilkins, Baltimore

Letts RM (1968) Myositis ossificans progressiva. A report of two cases with chromosome studies. Can Med Assoc J 99:856–862

Levinsohn EM (1980) Computerized tomography of the musculoskeletal system. JAMA 244:278–280

Lindenbaum RH, Clarke G, Patel C, Moncrieff M, Hughes JT (1979) Muscular dystrophy in a X;1 translocation female suggests that Duchenne locus is on X chromosome short arm. J Med Genet 16:389–392

Lindstrom JM, Seybold ME, Lennon S, Whittingham S, Duane DD (1976) Antibody to acetylcholine receptor in myasthenia gravis. Neurology (Minneap) 26:1054–1059

Lipicky RJ (1979) Myotonic syndromes other than myotonic dystrophy. In: Vinken PJ, Bruyn GW (eds) Handbook of clinical neurology, vol 40. North-Holland, Amsterdam New York, pp 533–571

Lutterbeck EF (1972) Die Bedeutung der Mammographie und Xeroradiographie zur Früherkennung des Brustkarzinomas. Zentralbl Chir 97:713–719

Lynas MA (1956) Dystrophia myotonica with special reference to Northern Ireland. Ann Hum Genet 21:318–338

Mabry CC, Roeckel IE, Munich RL, Robertson D (1965) X-linked pseudohypertrophic muscular dystrophy with a late onset and slow progression. N Engl J Med 273:1062–1070

MacCullough EC (1977) Factors affecting the use of quantitative information from a C.T. scanner. Radiology 124:99–107

MacCullough EC, Payne JT (1978) Patient dosage in computed tomography. Radiology 129:457–463

Major P, Resnick D, Greenway G (1980) Heterotopic ossification in paraplegia: a possible disturbance of the paravertebral venous plexus. Radiology 136:797–799

Markand O-N, North RR, D'Agostino AN, Daly DD (1969) Benign sex-linked muscular dystrophy. Neurology (Minneap) 19:617–633

Mategrano VC, Petasnick JP, Clark JW, Bin AC, Weinstein R (1977) Attenuation values in computed tomography of the abdomen. Radiology 125:135–140

Maunder CA, Dubowitz V (1977) Electronmicroscopic X-ray microanalysis changes in calcium and phosphorus in dystrophic human muscle. Excerpta Med Int Congr Ser 343:108–116

Mauro A (ed) (1979) Muscle regeneration. Raven, New York

McComas AJ (1977) Neuromuscular function and disorders. Butterworth, London

McKusick VA (1978) Mendelian inheritance in man. Catalogs of autosomal dominant, autosomal recessive and X-linked phenotypes, 5th edn. John Hopkins University Press, Baltimore London

Melot GJ (1941) Roentgenologic examinations of the soft tissues; technical considerations; study of the axillary region. AJR 46:189–196

Meschan I (1978) Synopsis of radiologic anatomy with computed tomography. Saunders, Philadelphia London Toronto

Meyer AEFH, Elias EA (1976) The value of enzyme histochemical techniques in classifying fibre types of human skeletal muscle. Histochemistry 48:257–267

Miller LF, O'Neill CJ (1949) Myositis ossificans in paraplegics. J Bone Joint Surg [Am] 31:283–294

Mokri B, Engel AG (1975) Duchenne dystrophy: Electron microscopic findings pointing to a basic or early abnormality in the plasma membrane of the muscle fiber. Neurology (Minneap) 25:1111–1120

Moore RB, Appel SH (1980) Methylation of erythrocyte phospholipids in patients with myotonic and muscular dystrophy. Exp Neurol 70:380–391

Moser H, Wiesmann V, Richterich R, Rossi E (1964) Progressive Muskeldystrophie. VI. Häufigkeit, Klinik und Genetik der Duchenne-Form. Schweiz Med Wochenschr 94:1610–1621

Motta J, Guilleminault C, Billingham M, Barry W, Mason J (1979) Cardiac abnormalities in myotonic dystrophy. Electrophysiology and histopathologic studies. Am J Med 67:467–473

M.R.C. (1943) Medical Research Council war memorandum, no 7: Aids to the investigation of peripheral nerve injuries. HMSO, London (reprinted 1960)

Munsat TL (1979) The classification of human myopathies. In: Vinken PJ, Bruyn GW (eds) Handbook of clinical neurology, vol 40/I. North-Holland, Amsterdam New York Oxford, pp 275–293

Naidich TP, Pudlowski RM, Leeds NE, Deck MDF (1978) Hypoglossal palsy: computed tomography demonstration of denervation hemiatrophy of the tongue associated with glomus jugulare tumor. J Comput Assist Tomogr 2:630–632

Nemours-Auguste S (1959) Radiographie des parties molles à voltage élevé. J Radiol Electrol 40:319

Nesbit D, Levine E, Neff JR (1981) Direct longitudinal computed tomography of the forearm. J Comput Assist Tomogr 5:144–146

Newark H, Forrester DM, Brown JC, Robinson A, Olken SM, Bledsoe R (1978) Calcific tendinites of the neck. Radiology 128:355–358

Nihei K, Kamoshita S, Atzumi T (1979) A case of Ulrich's disease. Brain Dev 1:61–67

Nuttal FQ, Barbosa J, Gannon MC (1974) The glycogen synthase system in skeletal muscle of normal humans and patients with myotonic dystrophy. Effect of glucose and insulin administration. Metabolism 23:561–568

O'Doherty DS, Schellinger D, Raptopoulos V (1977) Computed tomographic patterns of pseudohypertrophic muscular dystrophy: Preliminary results. J Comput Assist Tomogr 1:482–486

Ogilvie-Harris DJ, Hous CB, Fornasier VL (1980) Pseudomalignant myositis ossificans: heterotopic new-bone formation without a history of trauma. J Bone Joint Surg [Am] 62:1274–1283

Oliphant WD (1955) Xeroradiography. 1. Apparatus and method of use. Br J Radiol 28:543–544

Olson ND (1978) Peripheral neuropathy in myotonic dystrophy. Relation to glucose intolerance. Arch Neurol 35:741–745

Orndahl G, Kock NG, Sundin T (1973) Smooth muscle activity in myotonic dystrophy. Brain 96:857–860

Osterman FA Jr, Zeman GH, Gopola UVR, Gayler B, Kirk BF, James AE Jr (1977) Negative-mode soft-tissue xeroradiography. Radiology 124:689–694

Otto RC, Pouliadis GP, Kumpe DA (1976) The evaluation of pathologic alterations of juxtaosseus soft tissue by xeroradiography. Radiology 120:297–302

Padykula HA, Gauthier FG (1967) Morphological and cytochemical characteristics of fiber types in normal mammalian skeletal muscle. In: Milhorat AT (ed) Exploratory concepts in muscular dystrophy and related disorders. Excerpta Medica-Elsevier, Amsterdam, pp 117–128

Pálvölgyi R (1978) Über die Röntgenmorphologie der Veränderungen der Extremitätenmusculatur. Radiologe 18:469–474

Pálvölgyi R (1979) Roentgenmorphological muscle changes in anterior horn cell lesions. ROEFO 130:338–341

Pálvölgyi R, Bálint BJ (1979) Radiographic diagnosis of closed muscle and tendon injuries of the upper arm. Arch Orthop Trauma Surg 95:177–180

Pálvölgyi R, Gallai M (1979) Roentgenmorphological aspects of muscular pseudohypertrophy. J Neurol Sci 43:83–94

Pálvölgyi R, Gallai R (1980) Use of X-ray techniques to demonstrate electively increased damage to certain muscles in patients suffering from muscular diseases. ROEFO 133:58–62

Pálvölgyi R, Pentek Z (1977) Xeroradiographic demonstration of soft tissues of the extremities. Acta Morphol Acad Sci Hung 25:189–195

Pálvölgyi R, Pentek Z, Csanaky A (1977) Xero-radiography in the X-ray diagnosis of the soft parts of the extremities. Magy Radiol 29:293–303

Pálvölgyi R, Bálint BJ, Jozsa L (1979) The Ehlers-Danlos syndrome causing lacerations in tendons and muscles. Arch Orthop Trauma Surg 95:173–176

Panayitopoulos CP, Scarpalesos S (1976) Dystrophia myotonica. Peripheral nerve involvement and pathogenetic implications. J Neurol Sci 27:1–16

Pearce RG, Höweler CJ (1979) Neonatal form of dystrophia myotonica. Five cases of preterm babies and a review of earlier reports. Arch Dis Child 54:331–338

Pearson CM, Fowler WG Jr (1963) Hereditary nonprogressive muscular dystrophy inducing arthrogryposis syndrome. Brain 86:75–88

Peter JB, Barnard VR, Edgerton VR, Gillespie CA, Stempel KE (1972) Metabolic profiles of three fiber types of skeletal muscles in guinea pigs and rabbits. Biochemistry 11:2627–2633

Pette D (ed) (1980) Plasticity of muscle. Proceedings of a symposium held at the University of Konstanz, Germany, September 23–28, 1978. de Gruyter, Berlin New York

Pickard NA, Goldsmith BM, Gruener HD, Isaacs ER, Nance WE, Crawford RG (1979) Lymphocyte capping in carriers of Duchenne muscular dystrophy. N Engl J Med 301:724

Pleasure D, Wyszynski B, Sumner D, Schotland DL, Feldmann B, Nugent N, Hitz K, Goodman DBP (1979) Skeletal muscle calcium metabolism and contractile force in vitamin D-deficient chicks. J Clin Invest 64:1157–1167

Plishker GA, Gitelman HJ, Appel SH (1978) Myotonic muscular dystrophy: altered calcium transport in erythrocytes. Science 200:323–325

Pollock M, Dyck PJ (1976) Peripheral nerve morphometry in myotonic dystrophy. Arch Neurol 33:33–39

Pons H (1958) Exploration radiologique des tissues mous. Ann Radiol (Paris) 1:671–678

Prince FP, Hikida RS, Hagerman FC (1977) Muscle fibre types in women athletes and non-athletes. Pfluegers Arch 371:161–165

Prot J (1971) Genetic-epidemiological studies in progressive muscular dystrophy. J Med Genet 8:90–96

Ralls PW, Boswell W, Henderson R, Rogers W, Boger D, Halls J (1980) CT of inflammatory disease of the psoas muscle. AJR 134:767–770

Rash PJ, Burke RK (1978) Kinesiology and applied anatomy. The science of human movement, 6th edn. Lea & Febiger, Philadelphia

Reniers J, Martin S, Joris C (1970) Histochemical and quantitative analysis of muscle biopsies. J Neurol Sci 10:349–367

Reville WJ, Goll DE, Stromer MH, Robson RM, Dayton WR (1976) A Ca^{2+}-activated protease possibly involved in myofibrillar protein turnover. Subcellular localization of the protease in porcine skeletal muscle. J Cell Biol 70:1–8

Ringel SP, Carroll JE, Schold C (1977) The spectrum of mild X-linked recessive muscular dystrophy. Arch Neurol 34:408–416

Roach JF, Hilleboe HE (1955 a) Xeroradiography. AJR 73:5–9

Roach JF, Hilleboe HE (1955 b) Xeroradiography. JAMA 157:899–901

Roberts DF, Bradley WG (1977) Immunoglobulin levels in dystrophia myotonica. J Med Genet 14:16–19

Rose AL, Willison RG (1967) Quantitative electromyography using automatic analysis. Studies in healthy subjects and patients with primary muscle disease. J Neurol Neurosurg Psychiatry 5:403–410

Roses MS, Nicholson MT, Kircher CS, Roses AD (1977) Evaluation and detection of Duchenne's and Becker's muscular dystrophy carriers by manual muscle testing. Neurology (Minneap) 27:20–25

Rotthauwe HW, Kowaleski S (1965) Klinische und biochemische Untersuchungen bei Myopathien. Klin Wochenschr 43:144–163

Rotthauwe HW, Kowaleski S (1966) Gutartige recessive X-chromosomal vererbte Muskeldystrophie. Hum Genet 3:17–40

Russell RGG, Bisz S, Fleisch H (1969) Pyrophosphate and diphosphonates in calcium metabolism and their possible role in renal failure. Arch Intern Med 124:571–577

Russell RGG, Mühlbauer RC, Bisaz S, Fleisch H (1970) The influence of pyrophosphate, condensed phosphates, phosphonates and other phosphate compounds on the dissolution of hydroxyapatite in vitro and on bone resorption induced by parathyroid hormone in tissue culture and in thyroparathyroidectomized rats. Calcif Tissue Res 6:183–196

Sagel J, Distiller LA, Morley JE, Isaacs H (1975) Myotonia dystrophica: Studies on gonadal function using luteinizing hormone-releasing hormone (LRH). J Clin Endocrinol Metab 40:1110–1113

Sarmiento AH, Alba J, Lanars AE, Dietrich R (1975) Evaluating soft-tissue calcification in dermatomyositis with ^{99m}Tc-phosphate compounds: case report. J Neurol Med 16:467–468

Schadé JP (1978) Introduction to functional human anatomy. An atlas. Saunders, Philadelphia London Toronto

Schotland DL, Borrilla E, Wakayama Y (1979) Pathogenesis of muscle cell damage in dystrophies: morphologic aspects including freeze fracture studies. In: Aguayo AJ, Karpati G (eds) Current topics in nerve and muscle research. International Congress Series 455:29–38

Schott GD, Wills MR (1975) Myopathy and hypophosphataemic osteomalacia presenting in adult life. J Neurol Neurosurg Psychiatry 38:297–304

Schwartz O, Jampel RS (1962) Congenital blepharophimosis associated with a unique generalized myopathy. Arch Ophtalmol 68:52–57

Seigel RS (1980) Heterotopic ossification in paraplegia. Radiology 137:259

Shaw RF, Dreifuss FE (1969) Mild and severe forms of X-linked muscular dystrophy. Arch Neurol 20:451–460

Siegel BA, Engel WK, Derier EC (1975) ^{99m}Tc-diphosphonate uptake in skeletal muscle: A quantitative index of acute damage. Neurology 25:1055–1058

Silberstein EB, Bove KE (1979) Visualisation of alcoholinduced rhabdomyolysis: a correlative radiotracer, histochemical and electron-microscopic study. J Nucl Med 20:127–129

Skinner R, Smith C, Emery AEH (1974) Linkage between the loci for benign (Becker type) X-borne muscular dystrophy and deutan colour blindness. J Med Genet 11:317–320

Skinner R, Emery AEH, Anderson AJB, Foxall C (1975) The detection of carriers of benign (Becker type) X-linked muscular dystrophy. J Med Genet 12:131–134

Soule ABJr (1945) Neurogenic ossifying fibromyopathies. A preliminary report. Neurosurgery 2:485–497

Spies SM, Swift TR, Brown M (1975) Increased ^{99m}Tc-polyphosphate muscle uptake in a patient with polymyositis: case report. J Nucl Med 16:1125–1127

Spranger JW, Schinzel A, Myers T, Ryan J, Giedion A, Opitz JM (1980) Cerebro-arthrodigital syndrome: a newly recognized formal genesis syndrome in three patients with apparent arthromyodysplasia and sacral agenesis, brain malfunction and digital hypoplasia. Am J Med Genet 5: 13–24

Stalberg E, Trontelj JV (1979) Single fibre electromyography. Mirvalle Presse, Old Working, Surrey, UK

Steinert H (1909) Myopathologische Beiträge: I. Über das klinische und anatomische Bild des Muskelschwunds der Myotoniker. Dtsch Z Nervenheilkd 37:58–104

Steinfeld JR, Thorne NA, Kennedy TF (1977) Positive ^{99m}Tc-pyrophosphate bone scan in polymyositis. Radiology 122:168

Sulemana CA, Suchenwirth R (1972) Topische Unterschiede in der enzymhistologischen Zusammensetzung der Skelettmuskulatur. J Neurol Sci 16:433–444

Suzuki Y, Hisada K. Takeda M (1974) Demonstration of myositis ossificans by ^{99m}Tc-pyrophosphate bone scanning. Radiology 111:663–664

Swift TR, Brown M (1978) Tc-99m pyrophosphate labeling in McArdle syndrome. J Nucl Med 19:295–297

Termote J-L, Baert A, Crolla D, Palmers Y, Bulcke JA (1980) Computed tomography of the normal and pathologic muscular system. Radiology 137:439–444

Théodore C, Cornud F, Molas G, Gehanno P, Mendez J, Paologgi J-A (1980) Les manifestations digestives de la maladie de Steinert. A propos de 4 cas. Gastroenterol Clin Biol 4:556–559

Thompson JS, Kreel L (1979) The subtrapezial space. J Comput Assist Tomogr 3:355–359

Thomsen J (1876) Tonische Krämpfe in willkürlich beweglichen Muskeln infolge von ererbter psychischer Disposition (Ataxia muscularis). Arch Psychiatr Nervenkr 6:702–718

Torch WC, Reno NV (1980) Computerized tomography of muscle: a useful technique in the differential diagnosis and study of infantile hypotonia and a variety of neuromuscular disorders in children and adults. (Abstract 72 of ninth annual meeting of the child neurology society, Savannah GA, October 2–4, 1980). Ann Neurol 8:233–234

Tredici G, Coletti A (1978) Dystrophia myotonica and hypothyroidism. J Neurol 218:215–218

Trokel SL, Hilal SK (1979) Recognition and differential diagnosis of enlarged extraocular muscles in computed tomography. Am J Ophtalmol 87:503–512

Tünte W, Becker PE, Knorre G (1967) Zur Genetik der Myositis ossificans progressiva. Humangenetik 4:320–351

Tweeddale DN, Higgins GM, Wakim KG (1957) Attempts to produce myositis ossificans in the rat. Lab Invest 6:346–356

Vinken PJ, Bruyn GW (1979a) Diseases of muscle. In: Handbook of clinical neurology, vol 40, part I. Elsevier/North-Holland, Amsterdam New York

Vinken PJ, Bruyn GW (1979b) Diseases of muscle. In: Handbook of clinical neurology, vol 41, part I. Elsevier/North-Holland, Amsterdam New York

Visser de M (1981) Ziekte van Becker (Becker's disease). Thesis, University of Amsterdam

Vita G, Harris JB (1981) The uptake of ^{99m}technetium diphosphonate into degenerating and regenerating muscle. A correlative histological and biochemical study. J Neurol Sci 51:339–354

Wadia RS, Wadgaonkar SU, Amin RB, Sardesai HV (1976) An unusual family of benign 'X' linked muscular dystrophy with cardiac involvment. J Med Genet 13:352–356

Wald CD (1975) Myotonic dystrophy. – Sedative and anaesthetic management. Oral Surg 39:875–885

Walton JN, Warrick CK (1954) Osseous changes in myopathy. Br J Radiol 27:1–15

Walton JN (1964) Muscular dystrophy: some recent advances in knowledge. Br Med J 1:1271–1274

Walton Sir JN (1981) Disorders of voluntary muscle, 4th edn. Churchill Livingstone, Edinburgh London

Weiner MJ (1978) Myotonic megacolon in myotonic dystrophy. Am J Roentgenol 130:177–179

Weiss IW, Fisher L, Phang JM (1971) Diphosphonate therapy in a patient with myositis ossificans progressiva. Ann Intern Med 74:933–936

Wilkins KE, Gibson DA (1976) The patterns of spinal deformity in Duchenne muscular dystrophy. J Bone Joint Surg [Am] 58:24–32

Willison RG (1964) Analysis of electrical activity in healthy and dystrophic muscle in man. J Neurol Neurosurg Psychiatry 27:386–394

Willison RG (1966) Some problems in the diagnosis of primary muscle disease. Proc Soc Med 59:998–1000

Willison RG (1968) Quantitative analysis of the EMG. Electroencephalogr Clin Neurophysiol 25:401–412

Wilson JS, Korobkin M, Genant HK, Bovill EG (1978) Computed tomography of muskuloskeletal disorders. Am J Roentgenol 131:55–62

Wilson CR (1979) Determination in vivo of fat and muscle mass in obesity with quantitative CT. J Comput Assist Tomogr 3:858–859

Wohlfart G, Fex J, Eliasson S (1955) Hereditary proximal spinal muscle atrophy simulating progressive muscular dystrophy. Acta Psychiatr Scand 30:395–406

Wolfe JN (1969) Xeroradiography of the bones, joints and soft tissues. Radiology 93:583–587

Wolfe JN (1972) Xeroradiography of the breast. Thomas, Springfield, Illionois

Wolfe JN (1973) Xeroradiography: Image content and comparison with film roentgenograms. Am J Roentgenol 117:690–695

Wong P, Roses AD (1979) Isolation of an abnormally phosphorylated erythrocyte membraneband 3 glycoprotein from patients with myotonic muscular dystrophy. J Membrane Biol 45:147–166

World Federation of Neurology: Research Group on Neuromuscular Diseases (1968) Classification of the neuromuscular disorders. J Neurol Sci 6:165–177

Wrogeman K, Pena SDJ (1976) Mitochondrial calcium overload: a general mechanism for cell necrosis in muscle diseases. Lancet 1:672–674

Wynne-Davies R, Loyd-Roberts GC (1976) Arthrogryposis multiplex congenita: Search for prenatal factors in 66 sporadic cases. Arch Dis Child 51:618–623

Zatz M, Itskan SB, Sanger R, Frota-Pessoa O, Saldanka PH (1974) New linkage data for the X-linked types of muscular dystrophy and G 6 PD variants, colour blindness, and Xg blood groups. J Med Genet 11:321–327

Zatz M, Shapiro LJ, Campion DS, Oda E, Kaback MM (1978) Serum pyruvate-kinase (PK) and creatine-phosphokinase (CPK) in progressive muscular dystrophies. J Neurol Sci 36:349–362

Zellweger H, Hanson JW (1967) Slowly progresive X-linked recessive muscular
   dystrophy (type III b). Arch Intern Med 120:525–535
Zimmerli O, Moser H, Lattke F, von Matt B, Gerber H (1977) Die eugenische Bedeutung der Kopplung zwischen den Genloci für Dystrophia myotonica (M.
   Steinert) und ABH-Sekretor. Schweiz Med Wochenschr 107:327–335

Subject Index

Abdominal Computer Tomography

With the collaboration of G. Marchal,
G. Wilms
1980. 315 figures in 585 separate illustrations.
XI, 185 pages (Atlas of Pathological Com-
puter Tomography, Volume 2)
ISBN 3-540-10093-8

Clinical Computer Tomography

Head and Trunk
Editors: A. Baert, L. Jeanmart,
A. Wackenheim
1978. 414 figures, 2 tables. VIII, 261 pages
ISBN 3-540-08458-4

Computer Reformations of the Brain and Skull Base

By R. Unsöld, C. B. Ostertag, J. de Groot,
T. H. Newton
1982. 237 figures including 76 colored plates.
Approx. 245 pages
ISBN 3-540-11544-7

Computerized Tomography

Editors: J. M. Caille, G. Salamon
1980. 139 figures, 31 tables. XVII, 293 pages
(INSERM-Symposium, Bordeaux,
September 20 22, 1979)
ISBN 3-540-09808-9

Computerized Tomography – Brain Metabolism – Spinal Injuries

Editors: W. Driesen, M. Brock, M. Klinger
1982. 186 figures, 76 tables. Approx. 420 pages
(Advances in Neurosurgery, Volume 10)
ISBN 3-540-11115-8

Craniocerebral Computer Tomography

Confrontations with Neuropathology
With collaboration of D. Baleriaux, D. Crolla,
J. Dietemann, R. Dom, J. Flament, N. Heldt,
Y. Palmers, J. Termote
1980. 112 figures in 498 separate illustrations.
X, 130 pages. (Atlas of Pathological Computer
Tomography, Volume 1)
ISBN 3-540-09879-8

Mathematical Aspects of Computerized Tomography

Proceedings, Oberwolfach, February 10–16,
1980
Editors: G. T. Herman, F. Natterer
1981. VIII, 309 pages. (Lecture Notes in
Medical Informatics, Volume 8)
ISBN 3-540-10277-9

M. A. Meyers
Dynamic Radiology of the Abdomen

Normal and Pathologic Anatomy
2nd edition. 1982. 1006 figures (17 figures in
full color). XV, 396 pages
ISBN 3-540-90629-0

H. Pettersson, D. C. F. Harwood-Nash
CT and Myelography of the Spine and Cord

Techniques, Anatomy and Pathology
in Children
1982. 93 figures. 136 pages
ISBN 3-540-11322-3

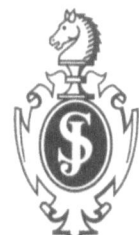

Springer-Verlag Berlin Heidelberg New York

Frontiers in European Radiology

Editors-in-Chief: A. L. Baert, E. Boijsen,
W. A. Fuchs, F. H. W. Heuck

Frontiers in European Radiology (FER)
addresses radiologists all over the world with
the goal of improving the international exchange of information on all aspects of radiological research. This exchange has unfortunately been limited in the past, especially by the
language barriers involved. As a result,
Europe's contribution to scientific progress in
this interdisciplinary specialty has influenced
only regional developments. A first step
toward rectifying the situation was taken in
Hamburg in September 1979, when the formation of the association of European
University Radiologists was discussed and
decided upon.

FER is the logical continuation of that initia-
tive; it will provide a forum for scientists in
European clinical and experimental radiology
where important reports on progress in the
field can be presented in a depth not possible
in a journal. It will be a concise source of
detailed information for those wanting to keep
abreast of the scientific progress in this field.

Volume 1

1982. 113 figures in 187 separate illustrations.
V, 170 pages
ISBN 3-540-10753-3

Contents:
I. Fernström, B. Johansson: Percutaneous
Extraction of Renal Calculi. – *R. Günther,
P. Alken:* Percutaneous Nephropyelostomy
and Endo-Urological Manipulations. –
*R. Pasariello, G. P. Feltrin, D. Miotto,
S. Pedrazzoli, P. Rossi, G. Simonetti:* Trans-
hepatic Portal Catheterization with Pancreatic
Venous Sampling Versus Angiography in the
Localization of Pancreatic Functioning
Tumors. – *G. M. Kauffmann, G. Richter,
J. Rassweiler, R. Rohrbach:* New Topics in
Embolization. Effects of Central, Peripheral
or Capillary Occlusion Type in Animal
Models Simulating Tumor Embolization. –
F. Brunelle: Electric Transcatheter Vascular
Obliteration: Electrothrombosis. Electrolysis
or Electrocoagulation. – *V. Hegedüs,
O. Winding, J. Grønvall, P. Faarup:* Manu-
facturing-Derived Impurities in Angio-
graphy. – *K.-H. Hübener:* Digital Radiography
Using a Computed Tomography Intrument.

Volume 2

1982. Approx. 83 figures, approx. 6 tables.
Approx. 112 pages
ISBN 3-540-11349-5

Contents:
W. Loeffler: NMR as an Imaging Method. –
R. E. Steiner, G. M. Bydder: Initial Clinical
Experience with NMR Imaging. – *F. W. Smith:*
NMR Imaging of the Liver and Kidney. –
P. Marhoff, M. Pfeiler: Digital Fluorography. –
*M. P. Capp, S. Nudelman, D. Fisher, T. W. Ovitt,
G. D. Pond, M. M. Frost, H. Roehrig, J. Seeger,
D. Oimette:* Digital Radiography. –
A. B. Crummy, C. A. Mistretta: Digital Subtrac-
tion Arteriography (DSA). – *T. F. Meaney,
M. A. Weinstein, E. Buonocore, J. H. Gallagher:*
Digital Subtraction Angiography: Cleveland
Clinic Experience.

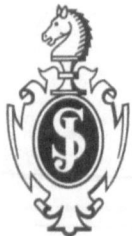
Springer-Verlag Berlin Heidelberg New York